LEADING CHANGE IN HEALTH AND SOCIAL CARE

Learning is at the heart of change. This book breaks new ground in exploring the need for individuals to engage in personal change through learning as an essential part of achieving significant change in organisations. It explains how to engage with people's energy, enthusiasm and abilities to enable them to think and do things differently.

Providing an overview of leadership theories and a practical guide to management tools and techniques, *Leading Change in Health and Social Care* is illustrated throughout with examples drawn from health and social care settings. Key topics covered include:

- contemporary models of transformational leadership;
- learning as the foundation of personal and organisational change;
- systems thinking as a way of understanding change in complex services;
- visions of a better future and how to develop them;
- values and how they influence our choice of direction;
- inspiring ourselves and others to take action.

This is a book for everyone who wants to improve health and social care services and enhance the experience of patients and service users. It assumes no previous knowledge of change management and is appropriate for students, teachers, trainers and professionals.

Vivien Martin works for the NHS as a member of the development team establishing the NHS University, an exciting new initiative in which learning is seen as central to improvement of the patient experience. She previously worked for the Open University Business School leading development of the NHS/OU distance learning material for managers in health and care.

LEADING CHANGE IN HEALTH AND SOCIAL CARE

Vivien Martin

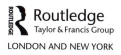
Routledge
Taylor & Francis Group
LONDON AND NEW YORK

First published 2003
by Routledge
11 New Fetter Lane, London EC4P 4EE

Routledge is an imprint of the Taylor & Francis Group

© 2003 Vivien Martin

Typeset in Futura and Sabon by
Florence Production Ltd, Stoodleigh, Devon
Printed and bound in Great Britain by
TJ International Ltd, Padstow, Cornwall

British Library Cataloguing in Publication Data
A catalogue record for this book is available from the British Library

Library of Congress Cataloging in Publication Data
Martin, Vivien, 1947–
Leading change in health and social care/Vivien Martin.
p. cm.
Includes bibliographical references and index.
ISBN 0–415–30545–4 – ISBN 0–415–30546–2 (pbk.)
1. Health services administration. 2. Social work administration.
3. Organizational change. 4. Leadership. I. Title.

RA971.M365 2003
362.1′068–dc21   2002037071

ISBN 0–415–30545–4 (HB)
ISBN 0–415–30546–2 (PB)

CONTENTS

FIGURES

EXAMPLES

INTRODUCTION

This book is for everyone who cares enough about our health and social care services to want to contribute to improving them. It is not only for those who are in senior positions but for anyone who can influence other people to generate enthusiasm for change. Everyone who works in or uses health and care services has the potential to lead change for improvement.

The focus is on leading change by developing commitment to achieving a better future. This involves people and their energy, enthusiasm, values and ability to think and to do things differently. If we don't learn to think and do things differently we will not change. Learning is at the heart of change. When we learn we make a change in ourselves, we increase our understanding and our potential to apply that new understanding to how we live and work.

Therefore this book presents an approach to leading change in health and care services that focuses on securing the willing involvement of colleagues and service users. It assumes that leaders can and do emerge from all areas of service provision and that leadership is shared and collaborative and not the sole responsibility of senior staff.

OVERVIEW OF THE CHAPTERS

The chapters are arranged to introduce this approach to leadership. Chapters 1 to 7 review ideas about leading and change in health and social care, including thinking, learning and acting as a leader and change agent. A model of the process of leading change is introduced in Chapter 1 and developed in Chapter 8. This provides the focus for the second group of chapters on being aware and focusing, developing vision and direction, inspiring action and reviewing, revising and reflecting. The final chapter discusses the nature of transformation.

Chapter 1 – Learning, leading and change in health and social care – asks why we need leaders when change is a normal part of life. The experience and process of change are discussed and a model of the process of leading change is developed to include learning and change processes.

Chapter 2 – The context of leadership – considers how our ideas about leaders have changed as we have become aware of the transformational nature of leadership and its processes in a social context.

Chapter 3 – Thinking as a leader – focuses on the different types of thinking that enable change agents and leaders to see things from different perspectives and to develop new approaches.

Chapter 4 – Learning to change – discusses how learning underpins personal change and the implications of learning to change in health and care settings. In particular, it focuses on learning that transforms people and the implications for those engaged in and leading transformational change.

Chapter 5 – Taking a leading role – begins by considering how people become leaders and what we expect of leaders. It goes on to consider how leaders can contribute to reducing levels of stress during change.

Chapter 6 – Developing change agents – is about developing individuals, groups and teams to be able to achieve change.

Chapter 7 – Leading learning – reviews how leaders can take an evidence-based approach to learning in an organisation and contribute to development of a learning culture.

Chapter 8 – Being aware – focuses on the first stage of the process of leading change by looking at what drives change and how change might be achieved in complex systems.

Chapter 9 – Finding a focus – develops the systems thinking approach to understanding the context of change.

Chapter 10 – Developing vision – focuses on how to develop a vision of a better future and explores both creative visioning and systems thinking approaches.

Chapter 11 – Developing direction – begins by discussing the extent to which values influence choice of direction and moves on to outline a traditional approach to planning although some concerns about planning are also discussed.

Chapter 12 – Inspiring action – is about inspiring others to take action to make the agreed changes and also about ways in which leaders might work with support and resistance.

Chapter 13 – Reviewing, revising and reflecting – is the last stage in the process and includes evaluating and learning from change. This may, of course, lead to increasing awareness of the need to change and a further journey round the cycle of change.

Chapter 14 – Transforming – stands back a little to reflect on transition and some of the very difficult issues that often need to be faced in transformational change. If these can be overcome, there is potential to achieve the better future that we can imagine for our service users and for ourselves.

CHAPTER 1

LEARNING, LEADING AND CHANGE IN HEALTH AND SOCIAL CARE

This chapter considers why change has become such an important part of our lives in health and social care and reviews the leadership roles that we all take in initiating and implementing change. Leading is essentially about visualising, understanding and progressing change. Leadership is crucial in contemporary health and social care to inspire people to make changes to improve services.

Staff and service users are acutely aware through their own experience of the speed of change in health and care services. Changing our ways of working usually means that we have to learn to think differently and learn to do things differently. People who understand how to facilitate learning can make an important contribution to change processes. Leaders who understand learning processes can approach change in a way that enables all those involved to learn as they engage in change.

This chapter concludes with a model that sets out the ways in which the book addresses learning, leadership and change in health and social care services.

LIVING WITH CHANGE

We are used to living with change. Change is natural in our universe. It is part of everything in our lives. We are all aware of how our bodies and minds change but, perhaps, less aware of the continuous change in things that change much more slowly, such as rocks, mountains and continents. News media make us all aware of change in the world through reports of natural disasters such as flooding, earthquakes and forest fires. We hear about ecological change including deforestation, climate change causing rising levels of sea water, and threats to our food supplies. We see change around us all the time through the seasons of the year. Even in inner cities we see constant change as communities come and go and buildings and resources are adapted. We also take initiatives to generate change ourselves.

'Those who believe in the continuity of this industrial age and seek to cling to patterns of work and life as we knew them are not going to license or encourage any exploration of new possibilities. It needs courage to admit that the old must go to give place to the new . . .' (Handy, 1985, p. 13)

Many workers in health and care services are tired of change and feel that they have been worn out by one initiative after another. Sometimes people in public services think that the pressure to change comes from change in government policies. This is true to some extent, but there are pressures that cause politicians to develop these policies. For example, if these services are seen as needing to respond to ever-increasing public demand, the capacity of services must increase and they will cost more to provide, so additional funding must be raised, probably through taxation. An alternative might be to try to reduce demand by educating citizens to take more care of their own health – but then different types of services would be needed to deliver support. As we develop greater technological expertise, different ways of treating illness and improving health become possible. As soon as new treatments and approaches become possible, information travels very fast (often through our improved electronic highways) and members of the public will expect health and care practitioners to know all about the latest methods and to be able to deliver them.

Our health and care services are like ships in a turbulent ocean of ever-changing movements and patterns. The waves on the surface make an immediate impact and we are often forced to change direction or change our speed to reduce the disruption. Storms or a change of climate in a specific location may even cause us to change our minds about where we are going, to choose a different direction. Currents beneath the surface may have a less directly observable impact on our progress but can have a significant impact on speed and direction. Rocks provide obstacles that can endanger us or cause us to change direction or to move carefully through channels that avoid contact. There is risk in most of our progress and, as everyone knows, ocean liners are very slow to stop or turn around. We need to maintain the ship to keep it afloat, to hold on to our sense of direction but also take care to navigate around obstacles and constraints. We also need to take advantage of the flexibility we have in our various situations if we are to adapt quickly enough to respond to changing circumstances. We need leaders to help us to take these initiatives.

WHY ARE LEADERS NEEDED?

Many environmental factors put pressure on organisations to change and we might be tempted to stand back and let whatever will happen just happen. This would be a reactive approach to change, where we formulate a response to each thing that happens, adapting to developments or trying to fix things that have gone wrong. The alternative approach is one of thinking and planning to predict the need to adapt or to try to prevent things from going wrong – a proactive approach. Most of us who care about providing reliable and high-quality services want to do everything possible to make sure that these services are delivered without hitches, so we favour taking a proactive approach. Proactive change in organisations and services has to be initiated and progressed by people. These people are leaders.

Leaders work with others to visualise how change could make an improvement, they create a climate in which the plans for change are developed and widely accepted and they stimulate action to achieve the change. Leaders who can work with others to achieve improvements are needed at all levels of health and care services. Leaders are needed to make the small day-to-day changes that ensure services continue to meet the changing needs of the communities they serve. Leaders are also needed to achieve the more dramatic step changes that have to be accomplished to change the direction or focus of services when new approaches are introduced.

THE EXPERIENCE OF CHANGE

Change is often discussed as though it is something abstract that will affect an organisation or service, but any change in these structures will have a personal impact on the people who work in them or use their services. Health and care services deliver many different types of care to large numbers of people, but in ways that attempt to meet their individual needs. These are personal services and people who use our services often feel frightened and vulnerable. Those who deliver and those who use services engage in them through interpersonal, face-to-face transactions. People learn to do things in particular ways and become accustomed to particular ways of doing things. Change involves doing things in different ways.

Change often requires people to think about things in a different way as well as to do things in a different way. This is one reason why change can be so difficult for individuals, particularly when people are feeling tired or anxious. Instead of going through the motions with familiar roles and activities, change requires an additional effort from us. In order to think and act differently, we have to learn new ways.

Health and care services are experienced in very personal ways both by staff and service users.

We are often frightened about having to learn and change, which is odd because we all have personal experience of successful dramatic change in our own lives. We all somehow learn to grow from being babies into adults, going through many different stages and somehow accepting that as we grow and change, we develop different views of the world. As adults we all have considerable experience of learning to change, but some of us have learnt to use processes that help us to learn from experience. Many practitioners in health and social care reflect on their experience of practice to help them to learn. Reflective practice is often based on the idea of an experiential learning cycle (see Figure 1.1).

Kolb and Fry (1975) viewed learning as a cyclical process with four key stages: concrete experience, observation and reflection, generalisation and abstract conceptualisation, with a final stage of active

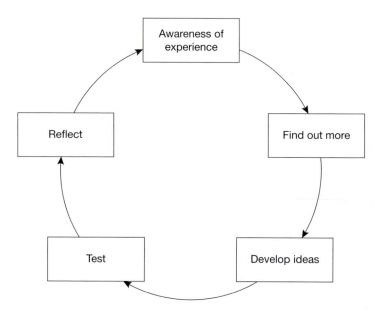

Figure 1.1   An experiential learning cycle

experimentation. In Figure 1.1 these stages have been described more in terms of what a learner does in the process of learning from experience. Kolb and Fry's final stage has been split into two, 'taking action' and 'reviewing'. The final stage of reviewing includes reflection, which often raises new questions and new ideas that provoke the learner to move once more around the learning cycle, so that it may become a perpetual process.

Stage 1, 'Awareness of experience', is the moment at which you realise you are experiencing something you do not fully understand. The learning process progresses to Stage 2, 'Find out more', where you look for more information to help you to understand the experience. You might do this by discussing the experience with others, observing others, reading about the issues or reflecting in other ways. When you have gathered enough further information, you are able to form some ideas or an understanding that seems to offer an explanation or a way forward. This is Stage 3, 'Develop ideas'. At this stage, the ideas are conceptual and so the next stage in the cycle is Stage 4, 'Test'. This is about trying out your new ideas in practice to see whether they solve the problem or puzzle or offer an explanation that sheds light on the experience. The final stage involves reviewing the extent to which the ideas worked when tried in practice and reflecting on how you might do things differently to achieve better results. This is Stage 5, 'Reflect'.

This sequence of recognising a concern, exploring and testing ideas and reflecting on what you have learnt can be applied to learning very straightforward things or to projects and investigations that involve much longer learning time-scales. Many practitioners in health and social care use this framework or a similar one in their regular reflection on practice to help them to ensure that they keep learning from their experience and avoid becoming complacent or rigidly repetitive in their practice.

LEADING A LEARNING PROCESS

As learning is so central to being able to change as an individual, an important element of leadership is the ability to facilitate learning. Leaders have their own learning processes and personal experiences of change as well as a potential role in encouraging others to develop understanding of the experiences that change brings.

Sometimes experience of change can be dramatic, even overwhelming, for individuals. Considering experience of this type as a learning process can help individuals to make sense of change for themselves. Although we learn constantly from day-to-day encounters, we are sometimes stunned to discover a completely new way of looking at things. Some call this experience 're-framing', derived from the idea of putting something in a new context or 'frame of reference'. For example, you might have had the experience of looking through the view-finder of a camera at a landscape but finding that as you move the camera you see elements of the landscape differently each time your focus changes and the boundaries move.

When individuals experience learning that is so significant that it represents a transformation in how they view themselves and their lives, this is 'transformational learning'. Transformational leadership is about achieving such significant change that situations are transformed and a new (and hopefully better) situation is created. The links between learning and leading change are close when the experience of those involved is considered.

Example 1.1:   Learning to change

Jack Mezirow describes some workplace learning initiatives that were designed to help people to think about new roles that they had taken as volunteer leaders. The programme was intended to develop the critical reflective ability of the volunteers to raise their awareness of their own attitudes towards many of the social issues that they would encounter in their work. There was a mixture of formal and informal learning situations and the learners found themselves changing their views about issues addressed by the agency, such as homosexuality, cross-cultural awareness and inclusive language. One of the volunteers said that the programme 'helped me to look at how we function and the roles we play out and how myths and stereotypes had shaped me and others. Up to then I had never looked at that, and to hear that, it made me take a look at myself and the traps I had been falling into'.
(Research by Trudie Preciphs discussed in Mezirow, 1991, p. 182)

In health and social care services there is wide understanding of reflective practice and experiential learning. This offers fertile ground for considering what type of leadership is appropriate in these interprofessional and interdisciplinary settings where people from disparate backgrounds contribute to service provision. Developing shared understanding and making meaning together are essential activities if learning and knowledge are to be captured and exchanged. There is increasing recognition of the need to encourage lifelong learning if people are to be able to keep up to date in our fast-changing world.

LEADING CHANGE IN HEALTH AND CARE SERVICES

We expect a lot from our leaders in health and care services. There has always been an expectation that senior people in professions, clinical and medical fields would offer leadership in developing their fields. More recently, staff in health and social care have been expected to contribute to the co-ordination of service delivery as it is configured in services and organisations. The structuring of work creates both bridges and barriers and can present obstacles that discourage staff from constructing the seamless service delivery that service users hope to find.

There is considerable evidence that indicates that we need to change and improve health and social care services urgently if they are to be able to serve us well in future. Social challenges are revealed in demographic changes that will require a different configuration of services to meet the needs of an aging population with expectation of longer quality of life. Citizens are becoming more demanding, wanting better information about matters that affect their health and welfare and also expecting greater involvement in decision making. Technology has improved the availability of information but also increases the demand on public services to ensure that appropriate information is made available in appropriate forms. Medical technology will continue to bring improvements to treatments and expectations will rise that the latest and best treatments will be available to everyone in need. The modernisation agenda in public services requires change to improve the quality of services so that the high standards achieved in some locations can be provided for every service user. Leaders from all areas of service delivery and from service users and user groups are the ideal people to identify local issues and to progress improvements in local collaborative initiatives.

To achieve the changes anticipated, leaders must emerge from all levels of services and from all service areas (see Example 1.2).

Example 1.2: Porters as leaders in developing seamless services

Max was a teamleader in the porterage services in a large hospital. He became very uncomfortable with the frequent informal complaints that were received, mostly about porters not being available when and where they were needed. He had been particularly upset by a recent episode in which an elderly man had used the hospital transport services to come for an outpatient appointment but had missed the bus for the return journey. The porters were accused of not returning to collect him, although there was no record of porters being asked to collect this patient, who had spent an uncomfortable and worrying period of several hours before anyone had noticed him and his distress.

Max decided that he could and would do something about this. He made informal approaches to the staff in each area of the hospital that regularly requested porters and asked them how they thought the service could be improved – what would they like porters to do that they don't do at the moment?

Max was astonished to find that no-one had asked them this before and that simply asking the question helped him to develop better relationships with many key individuals. He found that many things could be done to improve relationships and to improve the interface between the porters and each of the hospital services that porters work with. His approaches to individuals led to easier communication and to regular informal discussions about working together. He gathered stories about individual patients and how the porterage service had contributed to improving their experience of the hospital – and he shared these stories with his team. Soon he and his team became well known in the hospital as the porters who could get things done to help patients.

These leaders will need support to work confidently with their colleagues and service users to create local improvements. In addition, change in public services involves wider responsibility to a changing society, to promote inclusion policies and approaches, to insist on mutual respect and to emphasise equal opportunities. Leadership is a social activity, experienced and enacted through interpersonal relationships. Therefore the ability of a leader to inspire, motivate and support the activity of others is important, but carries responsibility in terms of the impact that change has on social groups.

Leaders who have enthusiasm and energy and who can inspire colleagues to support local initiatives will not necessarily be in positions that carry the necessary authority to progress change in organisations and structures. These people will have to be empowered by those who do have the authority and who can ensure that local initiatives fit harmoniously into the broad direction of the organisation or service area. Power and information have to be shared in empowering organisations and this is sometimes resisted in settings where hierarchical structures and authoritarian cultures are dominant. Empowered teams will be confident that their objectives support the

strategies of their organisations and services and will be supported
to achieve those objectives. Leaders in these teams will also have to
gain the confidence and support of colleagues who will be their fellow
teamworkers in achieving progress. Skilled problem-solvers who are
confident enough to assess and take appropriate risks can operate
effectively only if they are supported and empowered. We are increasingly aware of the interconnectedness of problems and solutions. It
is also important to keep an overview of the impact of change on
other service areas at the same time as paying attention to the detail
of particular initiatives.

In many areas of health and care services the prevailing organisational culture will have to change to encourage wider empowerment.
Culture change is not something that can be achieved by flicking a
switch – cultures develop through social interactions in fields of practice and everyone becomes aware in a multitude of subtle ways of
what types of thinking and what behaviours are broadly acceptable.
Those who act in ways not approved by the prevailing culture are
seen as challenging the majority, working in 'counter-cultural' ways
and generally causing trouble for people who are happy to leave
things as they are. This disapproval does not mean that everyone
thinks that things are good as they are, but that any disruption is
unwelcome. Change, however, cannot happen without some disruption. Leaders must recognise their role in preparing people for
the disruption of change and be prepared themselves to consider the
many ways in which progress towards an improvement, even one
that brings widespread benefits, impacts on individual lives and experience of work or of receiving care or treatment.

Leaders can play an important role in recognising and reducing the
anxieties and stress caused by constant change so that energy can be
focused on improving the quality of services for service users and the
quality of life for those who provide services. High-quality improvements cannot be achieved unless there is some consensus as to what
high quality means for those who use and deliver services. We need
to develop appropriate ways of working in partnership with other
agencies who contribute to the support and range of services that are
needed by service users during their journey from seeking help back
to independent or supported living. These agencies vary in many
dimensions (size, funding, public, private or voluntary status, national
or local) but have in common their focus on providing some aspect of
health or care service delivery. It is not easy to overcome the obstacles
presented by the differences, but these barriers must be challenged
if we are to genuinely improve the experience of service users. To
achieve patient/client-centred service provision we must involve and
empower service users, carers and their representatives to work with
us to develop accessible, convenient and appropriate services that are
considered to be of high quality by both users and providers.

High-quality provision has been achieved in many areas of services
through development of systems and practices that are understand-

ably defended when results demonstrate success. In order to develop partnerships, however, potential partners have to be prepared to change themselves to achieve even better outcomes together. Leaders from all levels of health and care services are the people who are and who will be initiating the development of more integrated and responsive services.

LEADING CHANGE AS A PROCESS

Change in health and care services is never a simple progression from A to B because it inevitably includes a huge range of complex services and because change is experienced personally by both service providers and service users. People have to learn to think and work differently, even to live a little differently. Leading and change are inextricably linked because of the personal and interpersonal experience of change.

Leaders are involved in developing awareness that change is necessary, in visualising the nature of change, in progressing the journey from one state to another and in taking ownership of the change so that it becomes the new 'normal' state. This can be described as a process, not very different from the process of learning from experience – see Figure 1.2: Leading change in health and social care. This diagram allows us to consider the leadership process as reflective practice. This is potentially helpful in the health and social care

Leading change as a process:

- Being Aware
- Developing Vision
- Developing Direction
- Inspiring Action
- Reviewing, Revising and Reflecting

bringing us back to awareness.

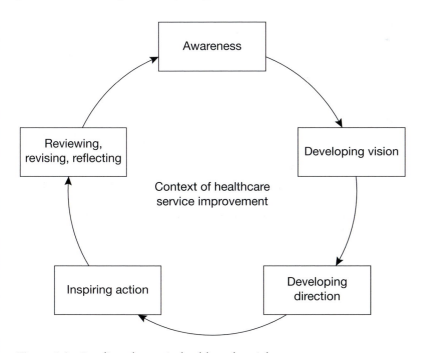

Figure 1.2   Leading change in health and social care

context as so many nurses, social workers and other professionals, clinicians, practitioners and managers use this basic reflective process to shape their continuing development in practice. Leaders emerge from all areas and levels of services and many may find it helpful to consider their approach to leadership in a way similar way to the approach they take to their practice in other roles.

The centrality of learning is acknowledged in Figure 1.2, where the experiential learning process is focused on improving the experience of the service user in the context of health and care services. The cycle is both the experiential learning cycle and the key stages in a change cycle.

The process outlined shows Stage 1, 'Awareness', as that in which a problem or puzzle is encountered (as in the experiential learning model) and the leader recognises that there is an opportunity to make an improvement. In Stage 2, 'Developing vision', the process involves both finding out more and developing a vision of a better future, usually with others who share concern about the issues. Stage 3, 'Developing direction', involves forming an understanding by making meaning from the information that has been gathered in the context of the particular problem addressed. At this stage the leader will also be developing ideas and plans that gain wide commitment from those who can help to make the vision a reality. In Stage 4, 'Inspiring action', the ideas and plans are tested in practice to progress in the direction that will achieve the vision. Stage 5, 'Reviewing, revising, reflecting', includes reviewing the results of the action, the opportunity to make revisions and time to reflect about what has been learnt. The review and reflection at Stage 5 may provoke a further journey around the cycle to amend or progress the change.

This chapter has introduced many of the ideas that shape this book. The approach to leadership is based on ideas that consider change and learning to be closely linked. This approach also expects leaders to be concerned with both achieving improvements with people willing to make changes and supporting those individuals through the learning processes provoked by the experience of change. Traditional and recent ideas about the nature of leadership are considered from this viewpoint, as is the nature of change. Further chapters explore the ideas that underpin different approaches to leadership and change and offer tools and techniques that can be used at different stages in leading a change process.

CHAPTER 2

THE CONTEXT OF LEADERSHIP

In this chapter we will consider some of the different ideas that have informed our thinking about leadership through the twentieth century and the ideas that challenge this thinking at the beginning of the twenty-first century. A number of theories that have been very influential in the past may still have something to offer us now. Much has been written about leadership, and the focus taken here is on considering how some of these classic theories relate to the context that we find ourselves in now in health and care services. Although these traditional theories were formed some time ago and in different contexts, they can still help us to understand more about how leaders think and act.

CHANGE IN PERSPECTIVE

Leadership used to be associated with the single heroic figure (usually a man) who was considered to be the inspiration behind an organisation, a military unit or a sporting team. This person was often seen as having superhuman abilities that enabled great victories to be achieved almost single-handedly. Those who contributed were seen as followers and teamwork was little appreciated.

We are now much more aware of the contribution made by everyone involved. In delivery of complex services no-one can deliver a high-quality service entirely alone. Teamwork is highly valued and we recognise that a person might play a variety of different roles in a team and also change roles frequently. This flexibility in teamwork includes flexibility about who takes a leading role and in what circumstances. Many organisations have become 'flatter' by reducing the number of levels in their hierarchies so that decision and action can be taken more quickly and by those who have direct contact with customers and service users. Flatter organisations, however, can only gain this speed of action if more people are involved in decision making and in initiating action. People at all levels and in all areas

> Leading at all levels – everyone is a potential leader.

of work are potential leaders and many organisations have taken steps to empower staff at all levels. The main issue in empowerment has been seen as ensuring that decision making is shared, so that only key decisions about organisational direction are taken at the most senior levels. This empowers those in all other parts of the organisation to make decisions that fit within the intentions of the organisation but closely meet the local needs and situations.

In health and social care services there is increasing awareness of the potential waste if staff are not empowered to work to their full potential. We recruit well qualified and competent staff who are costly to employ and it makes little sense to curtail their ability to work to their full potential by preventing them from using their judgement. There is, however, some concern about the extent to which we need to develop staff to be able to work to their full potential in empowered organisations. Those whose experience has been within the more sheltered environment of a single professional area of work, for example, may be able to make well informed judgements about matters within that familiar framework, but be less well informed about multi-professional environments where perspectives from the different professional viewpoints may differ. As we work more in multi-professional and interdisciplinary teams in health and social care we all need to learn to listen carefully to each other and to the patient or client involved when we have to contribute to decision making in complex situations.

In addition, wider recognition of the benefits of a diverse workforce has increased the range of different viewpoints and approaches in teamwork and leadership. Wider social inclusion increases the benefits offered by this diversity.

LEADERSHIP IN HEALTH AND SOCIAL CARE

In health and social care not only are our organisations hierarchical, but also the many professions that contribute to delivery of health and social care services have developed multi-layered hierarchies. Leaders are drawn not only from all levels of the various hierarchies but also from a wide range of clinicians, professionals and other practitioners. We might expect to see the number of layers in all of these hierarchies reducing to enable quicker and more local response to patient and client needs. In promoting services centred on service users, we should also expect much wider involvement of service users both as teamworkers and as leaders in developing new approaches.

For many years we have been concerned to enrich the multicultural mix in the health and social care workforce. Now that we are more conscious of the issues that arise in developing ways of working across and around traditional boundaries, the term 'multicultural' is increasingly applied to any work situation in which participants come from distinct groups that share elements of a distinct culture. For example, people from the same profession often seem to speak a language of their own and practitioners working in the same area of work can develop ways of thinking and acting together that are not easy for a newcomer to fit into.

Initiatives to modernise public services have brought waves of change. All the signs indicate that we need to learn to live with constant change. Many people find this exhausting although many others find it exhilarating. Health and social care services have very intense interpersonal relationships and how colleagues feel about what we are doing and experiencing has a strong influence on how service users experience the service offered. Leaders in all areas of service provision can influence the experience of both staff and service users and therefore can make a profound impression on how people feel about themselves, their experience and their well-being.

LEADERS AND MANAGERS

Leadership and management have been linked together, largely because there was wide concern in the 1990s about the roles that managers could play in developing more successful businesses and public services that met the needs of society more closely. This raised interest in the management of change which, in turn, brought a focus on the need for leadership.

Management roles have traditionally required managers to organise and control work, to plan, implement and review the effectiveness of work. This is usually within an established framework of structures and processes within an organisation. Leaders are linked more with change, hence might develop new systems and structures, new frameworks and directions. Therefore, although leaders do not have to be managers, managers are now often expected to demonstrate some leadership ability.

Kotter (1990) distinguished between management as being concerned with transactions and leadership as being concerned with transformation. Management roles involve planning, budgeting, organising, staffing, controlling and problem-solving, to create a degree of predictablity and order. Leadership roles are more concerned with establishing vision and direction, communicating the direction and aligning people, inspiring and motivating them and producing change.

Transactional and transformational roles.

A number of ideas, techniques and tools relating to management of change are equally relevant for anyone else leading change. Leadership and change are concerns for everyone, not only those in management roles. Change affects everyone and many people can and do take leadership roles. A more contemporary way of thinking about the relationship between managers and leaders is to think of both these roles as being 'added' to other roles. For example, a nurse, doctor, allied health professional, accountant, administrator or technician might all take on an additional role as a manager. Each of these might also take a leading role in progressing an improvement or change. Each might also be a member of several teams in which they take roles related to their expertise, experience or interests.

Leadership has fascinated people as long as groups have attempted to achieve a particular purpose. As early as the first century Pliny wrote about leadership in Roman military initiatives and Machiavelli's analysis of leadership in the wars between Italian Renaissance city states is still popular reading. In the early part of the twentieth century industrial developments fostered an interest in the nature of work and the potential both to improve working conditions and to increase output and profits. Here we review some of the early theories about leaders and leadership.

TRAIT THEORIES

Many studies were carried out in the first half of the twentieth century to try to identify the 'traits' that were common to famous leaders. This approach was based on the idea that it is personality and personal qualities that differentiate effective leaders from everyone else – that leaders are born and not made – that a certain set of personal characteristics determined who would become successful leaders. These are generally known as 'trait theories'.

Example 2.1:   Trait theories of leadership

Ideas about leadership in the early part of the twentieth century were based on the belief that leaders were born to the role. Many psychological studies attempted to identify what successful leaders had in common, but the number of characteristics, qualities and attributes proposed became too great to have any useful meaning. Traits that were consistently found included high energy levels, tolerance of stress, integrity, self-confidence and emotional maturity. It also became apparent that the situation in which leadership was demonstrated was important, as in some situations it was not possible to lead unless you were an experienced practitioner and able to command the respect of the group.

Early trait theory was rejected partly because of the impracticability of reviewing the range of characteristics proposed, but also because of the implication that if leadership was only a result of birth then it was the birthright of some privileged people and not of others. This belief implied that leaders could not be developed. Adair discussed trait theory as including a need to have a distinct personality and proposed that an important aspect of this would be integrity. He described integrity as 'wholeness', 'the type of person who adheres to some code of moral, artistic or other values' (Adair, 1983, p. 12). Studies found that the situation in which a leader was operating was also very important and that successful leaders often needed to balance one trait against another to accommodate the issues in the situation (van Maurik, 2001, pp. 4–6)

Many people rejected trait theories because of the implication that leadership is the right of those with inbred superiority. It is also possible that traits might be demonstrated by leaders because of the situations that they find themselves in rather than because of their personal make-up. The characteristics exhibited by leaders might therefore be considered to be more a behaviour than an inborn ability.

BEHAVIOURAL THEORIES

When trait theories seemed not to be providing acceptable answers about how effective leaders were produced, researchers began to study the behaviour exhibited by leaders. Behavioural theories are based on the idea that leadership is largely a matter of learning to display appropriate behaviour. Tannenbaum and Schmidt (1958) suggested that a person could choose a leadership style from a continuum that ranged from 'manager-centred' leadership through to 'subordinate-centred' leadership. This continuum demonstrates the tension between use of authority by a manager and the freedom of action allowed to subordinates.

Example 2.2:   Tannenbaum and Schmidt's leadership styles

Tannenbaum and Schmidt studied leadership styles in the 1950s. They expressed their results as a continuum ranging from manager-centred leadership (where authority was based on a traditional line management system) to the degree of freedom allowed to subordinates in this system. Seven positions were identified, broadly described as:

1. Tell (announce a decision and expect everyone to act accordingly).
2. Sell (explain the decision but do not invite discussion).
3. Discuss (present the decision and invite questions).
4. Negotiate (present a tentative decision subject to change after discussion).
5. Consult (present problem for discussion and sharing of ideas before the leader makes the decision).
6. Delegate (leader defines limits to enable decisions to be made by team members).
7. Collaborate (shared decision making and monitoring of progress).

Tannenbaum and Schmidt did not push this idea to its extremes, to suggest that a leader could have absolute authority or that authority could be completely abandoned – a style that might be considered abdication.
   (You can read more about these ideas in van Maurick, 2001, pp. 9–11.)

In management and leadership development all of these styles are considered to be potentially useful ones to adopt, depending on the particular circumstances. For example, in an emergency it is often appropriate for a leader to 'tell' so that action can be taken quickly. Similarly, a 'sell' approach might be appropriate when a decision has to be made by the person with appropriate responsibility and others have to be persuaded to comply. Other styles usually take longer, as they are more concerned with reaching agreement before action is taken. This is more important when team members need to be able to take action in an informed and committed way. Contemporary approaches to empowerment of staff at all levels put emphasis on leadership styles that explain issues and involve people in developing understanding of the options and the implications of choices that could be made.

A different approach to choice of styles was taken by Blake and Mouton in their model of the Management Grid in 1962. Their work developed the emerging idea that leadership styles varied in two important dimensions, concern for people and concern for achievement of the task. People-oriented leadership styles concentrated on good working relationships and the well-being of staff. Task-oriented leadership styles focused on setting goals and planning activities to ensure that the task was successfully completed.

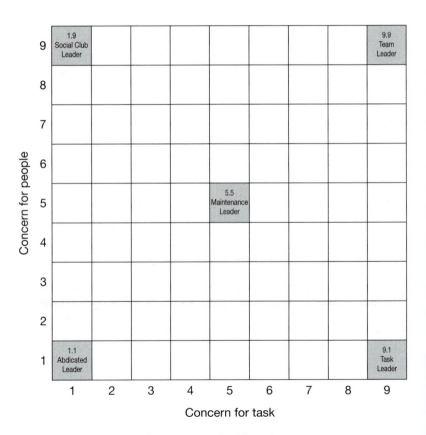

Figure 2.1   A style grid for leaders in health and care

Example 2.3:   A style grid for leaders in health and care

The style grid for leaders in health and care (Figure 2.1) uses two dimensions; the horizontal one is concern for task and the vertical one concern for people. There are nine points on each scale where 1 equals high concern and 9 equals low concern.

There are five descriptions of leadership styles that can be equated with squares positioned in this grid and the other squares allow you to identify a position that is less extreme than these key positions.

The position at 1.9 (concern for people very high and concern for task very low) indicates a type of 'Social Club Leader' where lack of conflict and general well-being are considered more important than achievement of tasks. This is often a popular style of management with staff and service users in situations where the achievement of task is less critical, perhaps in a long-term care situation as opposed to an Accident and Emergency setting in which this style would be very inappropriate. At the other extreme, 9.1, where concern for task is high and concern for people low, we find a 'Task Leader' where people are expected to perform as machines whose only purpose is to complete the task and the leader's responsibility is to plan, supervise and control the work. There are critical times in emergencies when this style is appropriate, but if this style is used for very long, people begin to feel as though they don't matter as individuals. For example, in an ambulance service there are times when quick and efficient action with little or no discussion is essential and other times when it is important to discuss incidents from every perspective so that lessons can be learnt and applied in future.

The other corners also represent extreme positions. At 1.1 is 'Abdicated Leader' where lack of effort expended on either people or task leaves an absence of leadership in which there is little motivation for people to work and where lack of decision making encourages conflict or indifference at work. This situation might be found if there has been no lead for some time and people feel unable to take a lead themselves. The opposite corner, 9.9, 'Team Leader', is often considered the ideal style to adopt with high concern for both people and task. This position should represent commitment to a common purpose and achievement through involvement and participation. With high concern for people, the service user would be the focus of interpersonal relationships and communication would be emphasised. The position in the middle, 5.5, 'Maintenance Leader', is the middle-of-the-road position where there is some attempt to achieve the task but with only moderate effort from the workforce. This might happen when everyone is tired after a major effort and represents maintenance rather than progression. This may be a politically expedient position to adopt from time to time, but the emphasis is on maintaining balance rather than making any change or progress. A position that is closer to continuous improvement is 7.7 where more attention is paid to both people and tasks but the tasks might be of a routine steady improvement nature.

(You can read more about these ideas in Pugh and Hickson, 1989, pp. 162–166.)

Another approach that still has resonance for us in contemporary experience of life in organisations is McGregor's theory of X and Y styles of managing work. Although these ideas were developed in relation to management style, they have been influential in consideration of choices of leadership style.

Example 2.4:   X and Y styles of managing work

McGregor's Theory of X and Y management (1960) contrasted two ways of working with people in terms of which approach produced better results. These approaches were an autocratic and directive style, Theory X and a participative style, Theory Y. These styles were based on different sets of assumptions about people and what motivates people.

Basic Theory X assumptions:

- people dislike and try to avoid work;
- therefore they need to be controlled with rewards and punishment to ensure that tasks are achieved.

Basic Theory Y assumptions:

- work is a natural activity and people like to commit themselves to achievement of tasks;
- the satisfaction of completing work well is a reward.

Those adopting Theory Y assumptions also think that work is often organised in ways that do not enable people to use their full intellectual or creative potential.

In many ways these positions can be aligned with the difference between autocratic managers who fear loss of control and democratic managers who lead by sharing and engaging others and who are able to risk loss of control by trusting others to be responsible. Many of the features of Theory X style are evident in contemporary organisations simply as a result of the ways in which administrative structures are developed to enable control of work. Theory Y proposes that people will find work more fulfilling and achieve better results if work is organised to enable inclusive and supportive relationships in which individuals can commit themselves to the objectives of the organisation. The tension between central control and local decision making is one feature of how we experience these opposing styles in contemporary organisations.

(You can read more about these ideas in Pugh and Hickson, 1989, pp. 156–161.)

Consideration of different types of behaviour in different circumstances led to thinking about the importance of the context of leadership, the situation in which a leader operates. These are generally grouped together as 'contingency' theories.

CONTINGENCY THEORIES

One of the main criticisms of behavioural theories was that they failed to acknowledge the importance of differences in situations. Contingency theories of leadership focused on the flexibility of a leader to choose and adapt an approach in response to different situations – contingencies. One of the earliest theorists was Fiedler (1967) who argued that both task- and people-oriented styles might be appropriate in different circumstances and that the effective leader chooses an appropriate style according to the demands of the situation. He identified three elements that indicate whether the situation is favourable to the leader:

■ whether the leader is liked and trusted by group members;
■ whether the task is clearly defined and well structured;
■ the power the leader has to reward and punish subordinates.

He found that a situation is very favourable to the leader when all three of these elements are strong. He also found that task-oriented leaders performed best in situations that were either very favourable or very unfavourable. Leaders whose style was more people-oriented performed better when situations were moderately favourable. Importantly, his work emphasised that the performance of the leader depends as much on the situation as on the style of the leader.

Fiedler thought that it was difficult for a person to change his or her leadership style but that it was possible to change the favourableness of a situation. This might be possible by, for example, increasing the authority and power of the leader or improving the structure and clarity of the task. Hersey and Blanchard (1988) disagreed with this idea and proposed that effective leaders should change their styles and should be able to adapt to the situation as they find it.

John Adair has been very influential in his contributions to thinking about both management and leadership. One of his key ideas was that a leader has to consider three sets of needs in approaching a task. These are the needs of the task itself, the needs of the group or team that is working on the task and the needs of the individuals who make up that group. His simple diagram of three focal areas in a leading role (see Figure 2.2) has been very helpful for people seeking a way of structuring their approach to a new situation.

Adair's model focuses on what a leader has to do in relation to the needs of each of these three areas. The first area, achieving the task, requires a clear understanding of the task and what success will mean. There will also be issues associated with the nature of the task, including need for information and maybe materials and equipment. The development of the team will normally include forming, developing and maintaining the team. The development of individual team members will include ensuring that individuals feel able to perform

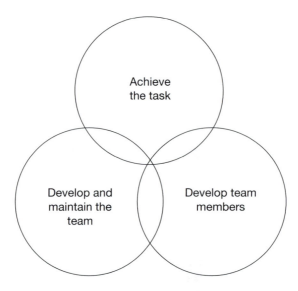

Figure 2.2   The leading role (adapted from Adair, 1983, p. 44)

in the team and development in relation to the context and task. Adair gives a full discussion of the issues in each of these circles and suggests that the relationship a leader might take to each circle is 'half-in and half-out' (Adair, 1983, p. 45).

Both behavioural and contingency theories have limitations. Most of them equate leadership with management and assume that this one senior person has power and authority over a number of subordinates. As organisations become less hierarchical these theories offer little to help us think about leadership amongst colleagues and in groups where roles frequently change. These theories are also focused more on the behaviour of leaders and the activities involved in completing tasks than the strategic direction and sense of purpose needed to achieve goals. Even the use of the term 'goal' is revealing, as some of our ideas about leadership have emerged from sports coaching.

TRANSFORMATIONAL LEADERSHIP

Leading change is about achieving a transformation – transformational leadership. Learning is fundamental in making transformations and therefore learning is an essential concern of leaders.

Earlier thinking – trait, behaviourist and contingency – is all about actions and transactions. The next wave of thinking was more about the nature of change, and leadership came to be considered as the ability to achieve a transformation. This is why we now associate leadership with change. Warren Bennis (discussed fully in van Maurik, 2001, pp. 99–107) was one of the earlier writers who associated learning with leadership. He thought that leadership could be learnt and that because learning is about taking control of your own life, learning is key to making transformations. In his view, the individual who can learn through reflection and who is able to make personal transformations is well equipped to translate this into achieving action and results in a wider context.

The main focus in ideas about transformational leadership is on people and change as something achieved by people. Peter Senge (1990) brought a valuable contribution to thinking about transformational leadership in his proposal that there are five essential disciplines that underpin organisations that are successful in learning from experience and transforming themselves to be effective in changing situations. These disciplines are:

- systems thinking;
- personal mastery;
- mental models;
- building shared visions;
- team learning.

These ideas are explored in more detail in other chapters in this book because they are influential in our thinking about both personal development as a leader and development of effective learning organisations.

There is also interest in the ways in which others perceive the behaviour of leaders, as this may shed light on what behaviours are considered successful in health and care services. Beverly Alimo-Metcalfe and Robert Alban-Metcalfe carried out a large-scale research study to identify the constructs that people in public and private services held about people that they considered to be leaders (Alimo-Metcalfe and Alban-Metcalfe, 2002, pp. 26–27). Constructs are mental models that people use to differentiate one leader from another, hence express what people consider to be important characteristics of leaders in public services. Some key factors of successful leaders were identified:

- concern for others;
- approachability;
- encouraging questioning and promoting change;
- integrity;
- charisma;
- intellectual ability;
- ability to communicate, set direction, unify and manage change.

Interviews with people in the public sector cited integrity much more often than those in private organisations. Sensitivity to the organisation's various stakeholders was also mentioned much more frequently by those in public services. This work underpinned the development of a diagnostic instrument to assess the behaviour and qualities of transformational leadership.

The linking of leaders to change, however, has challenged ideas that leadership can be objectively analysed and defined because there is so great an emphasis on people and the reactions of people to other people. As Grint observed:

> it is not that leaders are those who identify the wave and ride it; rather, leaders are those who persuade us a wave is coming, who go out of their way to appear the most visible surfers to onlookers, and whose actions are taken by the onlookers as actions appropriate for leaders to take.
>
> (Grint, 1997, pp. 9–10)

In the 1990s people began to think about leadership as a process in a social context.

LEADING AS A SOCIAL PROCESS

Leaders cannot exist without others, those who follow the lead. Following a leader implies more than simply doing what is asked, because leaders are asking people to commit themselves to making changes that will, potentially, have individual and collective impact. Once people agree to follow a lead, they become central to the process. Grint comments:

> If we argue, then, that leaders are those who in some way embody, articulate, channel and construct the values and direction that the followers think they ought to be going in, then we dispense with the leader as isolated hero and return to the leader as the embodiment of the collective.
>
> (Grint, 1995, p. 148)

If we follow this thought we realise that for a leader to be at all influential or effective, there must be a collective view of the direction of change. This requires an increasing emphasis on development in our organisations of an egalitarian social model that demonstrates social inclusion and intercultural approaches.

There are some important implications in the process view of leadership:

- A leader influences how people think about issues but he or she does not necessarily have formal power within an organisation.
- A group can have more than one leader – all members of a group can make leadership contributions. In 'dispersed' leadership, different people may demonstrate leadership in different areas. For example, different leadership abilities are required to develop strategy, develop team commitment and morale and to progress detailed tasks.
- If everyone is to be involved in committing themselves to change, everyone needs to know something about the impact of forces in

the wider environment surrounding our organisations and our work and understand why change is necessary to respond to these forces.

We need to consider development of all employees as potential leaders. In public services, we may also be concerned to involve service users in our teams as we develop our understanding of the need to change and become committed to progressing directions.

Those who have been working in health and care services are sometimes sceptical about the contribution that leaders can make in achieving improvements to service provision. In writing about nurses as leaders Colleen Wedderburn Tate comments:

> As the 21st century comes tip-toeing into life, the debate about leaders and leadership becomes more intense. But with all this talk, who has time to lead? The trouble is, leaders make us feel uneasy. After all, they are lauded, rewarded, and accorded all kinds of powers. We 'ordinary people' who like nothing better than to see the powerful get their comeuppance, make suitably disgusted noises, while firmly denying that we have a hand in the events we so roundly criticize.
>   . . . every healthcare worker has a responsibility to lead and exercise leadership. The fact that we may choose not to do so does not lessen our responsibility.
>
> (Wedderburn Tate, 1999, p. x)

If leaders are to be encouraged to emerge from all levels and all areas of health and care organisations, we must develop ways to identify and support the ideas that people propose. Some of our organisational structures will have to change to enable this diffusion of leadership activities and responsibilities through different areas of work. We might expect to find a need for different patterns of leadership for different parts of the organisation. Teamworking will need to be open to leadership coming from those who can inspire confidence to take action over a particular initiative rather than those in the most senior posts. We might expect our values to be frequently challenged and sometimes to be revised or reinterpreted to be more inclusive of the concerns of increasingly diverse groups and teams. The thinking and actions of teamworkers and leaders will fit the context, both the organisational environment and the culture. Power, responsibility and decision making will not be invested in one person but shared within a group. Leadership will be increasingly understood to be a dynamic process that includes and impacts upon people and progresses with a particular purpose.

In this chapter we have reviewed some of the most influential ideas about leadership. We have traced the changes in these ideas from the model of a heroic and probably male leader to ideas about leadership that are more inclusive and more contextual. If we agree that we need to develop more leaders at more levels in health and social care, we can note that there may be organisational constraints that must be addressed to facilitate able people to emerge. We may also need to find new ways of developing mutual understanding so that wide commitment can be achieved to enable progress towards change.

CHAPTER 3

THINKING AS A LEADER

In this chapter we consider how you can develop your own thinking and learning processes to ensure that they support you when you take leadership roles. We are very familiar with the experiences of thinking and learning but often have not made a conscious attempt to improve the ways in which we carry out these processes. First we consider why it is important to be aware of how we think and learn and how this connects to leadership and change. We then look more closely at ways of thinking that can support your development as a leader.

THINKING AND LEARNING

Thinking and learning are closely connected, but not the same. Thinking does not always lead to learning but is a process that we often carry out unconsciously in our day-to-day activities. We work things out and file them away as thoughts. Learning is more about making meaning from these thoughts, developing understanding that informs our thinking and actions. Learning is an essential component of change and thus of leadership.

Our familiarity with thinking and learning can be an obstacle if we simply assume that the processes are always working to support our own development. The processes associated with thinking and learning are similar because of the relationship between these mental activities. It is difficult to understand how someone else thinks or learns because the process is not visible, but the process can be shared and understanding developed collectively. Shared learning can be very important in developing understanding of perspectives brought by people with different experience. As an individual it is possible to become more aware of your own thinking and learning processes and to develop your own skills and abilities. As a teamworker or leader your awareness of thinking about approaches and learning approaches makes an important contribution to achievement of goals.

THINKING ABOUT THINKING

How do we think? I might say, 'I need time to think about that', before I feel ready to offer an opinion. What do I expect to do?

ACTIVITY 3.1

Allow 5 minutes.

If you say, 'I need to think about that', what will you do? Jot down three things that you might do.

1 _____
2 _____
3 _____

Our response to this invitation might be to run a mental search for anything we can remember about the issue. We might find some ideas in our own knowledge, or remember books or articles where we think there is more information. We might seek out people who we think know more about the issue than we do ourselves. When I say I want to think about something I usually mean that I want to find more information to help me to form an opinion. I might find out what opinions other people hold and why they formed those opinions. You might also have jotted down notes about particular ways of thinking, for example, creative thinking, thinking 'outside the box', being open-minded.

The first response to being asked to think about thinking might be 'Thinking is difficult!' The idea that thinking is difficult is often an old message from school that can be linked with failure if you were unable to remember something that you were supposed to have remembered. Memory is complicated because we store knowledge together with the 'tags' that we put on the things that we remember. These tags often incorporate our experience at the time when we 'stored' a particular memory. Thus as adults we are often stopped in our tracks by an old message that brings associations of failure and humiliation when we come across something that we were judged not to be good at as a child. These little gremlins are not easy to deal with, but the first stage in overcoming them is to notice them and to identify them as coming from you as a child rather than you as an adult. You as an adult can bring much more experience and self-knowledge to consideration of any particular issue. If you can put aside the memory that, for example, thinking was something that you didn't seem to do well as a child, you can approach it as an adult and ask yourself how you feel about it now.

IDEAS ABOUT THINKING AND KNOWLEDGE

Bohm (1994) suggested that thought and knowledge are collective rather than individual phenomena. Although we experience thought as personal and within ourselves, he felt that individual thought was largely the result of the individual's experience of making meaning from experience. The context in which we interact with others is made meaningful by the collective development of values, meanings and intentions. We create tensions and reactions as individuals within a collective:

> Each person is affected by the other people's thoughts, so that the reflexes of one person become the reflexes of the other. If one person is angry, the other is angry. It all spreads.
>
> (Bohm, 1994, p. 193)

Bohm also commented on the nature of knowledge. He challenged the idea that knowledge is ever permanent and absolute and proposed that there is nothing that we can consider permanently 'known'. He used his background as a physicist to give the example of the atom, which was originally thought to be something that couldn't be cut. Then later physicists found that atoms were made up of electrons, protons, neutrons and empty space – and then there were further discoveries (Bohm, 1994, p. 102). So knowledge is temporary and relative. It is a proposition that can be challenged as new understanding develops.

In some ways we acknowledge the temporary nature of knowledge when we use phrases such as, 'the current state of knowledge about . . .', or say 'we used to think . . .' when we realise that things have changed so much that it wouldn't be appropriate to think like that now. For many people, these ideas about thinking and knowledge seem rather slippery and alarming as we seem to be losing the solid ground on which we believe our knowledge to rest. How can we regard knowledge as transitory when so much of our technology, our disciplines and professions, our cultural traditions, our experience of life, appear to be firmly grounded in our collective knowledge? On the other hand, how can we not regard knowledge as transitory when we have experience of the impact of new discoveries, new ideas and developments arising from these?

If we accept that knowledge is transitory we must accept the possibility that our personal knowledge may be out of date. The knowledge that informed our actions five years ago might no longer be a sound basis for decisions today. This is not easy to accept,

'Almost daily, the headlines herald new advances in computers, telecommunications, biotechnology, and space exploration. In the wake of this technological upheaval, entire industries and lifestyles are being overturned, only to give rise to entirely new ones. But these rapid, bewildering changes are not just quantitative. They mark the birth pangs of a new era.' (Kaku, 1998, p. 4)

particularly if you feel that you have spent a long time memorising knowledge with the idea that it would inform your practice for the rest of your life. You might console yourself with the notion that the plethora of outdated knowledge that is stored away in your brain may provide a starting point from which you can check out current thinking and review the extent to which ideas have changed.

In health and social care, professionals, clinicians and others, whose work is informed by traditional bodies of knowledge, are increasingly aware of the need for continuous personal development. One area of development that is relevant to everyone in health and social care is the emergence of electronic databases that offer open access to knowledge that was formerly held in books, journals and libraries of professional bodies with restricted membership. Access to this knowledge used to be restricted to those who had the training to seek out and evaluate information as well as those who were able to gain physical access. Now many of the emerging databases are presented with an interpretation that is written in language accessible to the non-specialist and available to anyone who can access the world wide electronic network. We might note that although interpretations are often provided for us, there is still a need to make judgements if the information is to be applied. We might all be better informed about the nature of the judgement that has to be made but it still may be appropriate to consider who or what group are best equipped to make a judgement. Our personal and collective experience and knowledge define some of the differences that characterise the workforce in health and care services.

THINKING 'OUT OF THE BOX'

'When asked what they do for a living, most people describe the tasks they perform every day, not the purpose of the greater enterprise in which they take part. . . . They "do their job," put in their time and try to cope with the forces outside of their control. Consequently, they tend to see their responsibilities as limited to the boundaries of their position.' (Senge, 1990, p. 18)

We are often perceived to be rather limited and constrained in the ways we think – hence the frequent exhortation to think 'outside the box'. The 'box' is often the viewpoint that we adopt, often without realising it, that limits our breadth of thinking. We have to have these 'boxes' in order to survive day-to-day living. We simply don't have time to think about how to get up in the morning or how to cross a room, open a door and walk down a corridor – we just do these things on 'automatic pilot'. This automatic system is derived from our history. In the process of thinking we often refer only to our own history, the past experience that includes unconscious feelings, values and perceptions that we've stored away. The danger with limiting our thinking to this historically grounded approach is that nothing new can be easily accepted if it does not fit the old frameworks. We are tempted to discard new ideas and approaches if they seem to challenge our familiar world.

Argyris and Schon (1978) suggested that the sort of thinking that is limited to a single viewpoint and resists influence from wider perspectives is 'single-loop' thinking and is a closed process. They proposed a model of 'double-loop' thinking that is based on seeking out a wide range of viewpoints, taking an inclusive approach to discussion and monitoring implementation. This approach should be less defensive and provides opportunities for assumptions to be confronted and tested in a public forum. These more inclusive approaches have been widely adopted in health and social care services and we now expect to have wide consultation about significant change issues.

The problem that remains is that those who think in single-loop ways often do not realise that they are closing off the opportunity to consider other perspectives. Sometimes we head off into planning or decision making without checking whether we are running on 'automatic' or whether we should be disengaging to enable opportunities for different approaches to be considered. We are often resistant to considering a different approach, especially if there is time pressure or a general opinion that tried and tested methods are always the best. Consequently, many ideas have been offered both about how we might think more logically and about how we might think more creatively.

CRITICAL THINKING

Critical thinking is one approach to a more logical and structured way of thinking. Critical thinking implies logical reasoning, questioning of assumptions and ability to structure an argument. It also includes the ability to identify flaws, contradictions and ambiguities in lines of reasoning. The word 'critical' is not used in the sense of finding fault, but more in the sense of making a critical appraisal in which both positive and negative aspects are considered.

When we are faced with something we don't fully understand, it is easy to allow our thoughts to wander around, hoping that it will begin to make sense, perhaps even drifting off to think about something else. A critical thinking approach would be to recognise that you might become overwhelmed and to organise how you will structure your approach. You might decide what to focus on, how to identify the important features, what results you want to achieve, what steps you might take to achieve those results. A critical thinking approach is purposeful and structured. The structure is based on reasoning, a process that involves considering evidence and options in the context of certain criteria.

A critical thinker is able to ask questions and consider different perspectives and different possibilities in order to make her or his own judgements. In addition, a critical thinker will question the reliability of information and the way in which data and information are interpreted. On one level, this means being careful to check for accuracy and to ensure that all available information has been considered. It also means being self-aware and acknowledging one's own bias and limitations. A critical thinker is often considered an independent thinker, someone who is fair-minded and open-minded but who is able to seek and review evidence and form an opinion that can be explained and defended. A critical thinker is also able to evaluate the extent to which judgements can be based on the evidence that has been presented. In the complex workplace settings of health and social care it is very rare to feel absolutely certain that a judgement has been reached because everything that needs to be known is known and therefore the chosen solution is absolutely right. We usually have to base our judgements on 'weight' of evidence and confidence that alternative explanations have been considered and rejected.

Critical thinking approaches are increasingly important in our working lives as we are required to make decisions and judgements based on available evidence. Critical thinking skills include:

- taking a purposeful approach;
- asking focused questions;
- collecting and evaluating data and information;
- identifying potential for bias;
- distinguishing fact from possibility;
- identifying any assumptions;
- checking for accuracy and reliability;
- identifying any inconsistencies;
- considering alternative possibilities and explanations;
- assessing whether the evidence presented supports the conclusions claimed.

These are skills that everyone needs if they are to be able to question and evaluate the information that threatens to overwhelm all those whose work is necessarily informed by up-to-date evidence and research.

CREATIVE THINKING

Creativity is often problematic within structured organisational settings that rely on order and discipline to function effectively. The nature of creativity is to be different, often to challenge existing ways of thinking. Processes that encourage creative thinking can seem childish or subversive to those whose work normally requires them to be disciplined and compliant. In organisations that have valued compliance in the past there is often difficulty in changing and updating, as there is reluctance to change well established systems. These organisations find that they have to take steps to encourage the workforce to become more challenging and proactive so that improvements can be made.

Creativity is not as elusive as many believe it to be. It is often regarded as a gift that some have and some don't, that you are either born with or have to live without. There may be a measure of truth in this for those who demonstrate outstanding creativity, but for the vast majority of people, creativity is a forgotten ability that can be revitalised and nurtured. Most of us were able to play creatively as children. Somehow we lost the ability or forgot how to think in the creative ways we used to use. Sometimes we put our creativity aside if we are trained in logical thinking processes that seem to be more adult or more appropriate to the world of work. The more that we learn to value logical thinking above creative thinking, the harder it is to recover our creative abilities.

There are some processes that promote creative thinking. Many artists, musicians and other creative people use exercises to challenge, stretch and develop their creative thinking. Everyone else can do this too. Edward de Bono used the term 'lateral thinking' (1990, but first published in 1971). He offered a useful observation about why we find creative thinking difficult:

> The huge effectiveness of mind arises directly from the way it organizes information into patterns. The more firmly a pattern is established the more useful it becomes. But creativity involves breaking out of established patterns in order to look at things in a different way. Thus the very effectiveness of mind in establishing fixed patterns makes creativity very difficult. It is like having a filing system set up to store data in a particular way. In order to pursue cross-references in such a filing system, one would have to develop new ways of using it.
>
> (de Bono, 1990, p. 1)

De Bono proposed that the skill of lateral thinking could be learned and applied in order to be creative. He contrasted lateral thinking with vertical thinking, thinking that follows linear patterns such as building by placing one brick on another. He suggested that there are three stages in becoming able to think laterally (adapted from de Bono, 1990, p. 46):

- Develop an attitude towards change and towards new ideas.
- Escape from the inhibiting restrictions of vertical thinking.
- Develop techniques and tools.

De Bono and many others have suggested activities that help individuals and groups to escape from self-imposed restrictions in their thinking and that help to generate new ideas.

Example 3.1:   Challenging existing practices – developing an attitude towards change

This exercise can be done alone or with others. Start by making a list of all the things that you would like to happen in your organisation. Write them as though they are happening. For example:

■ We all try to offer the best possible service to each other so that we provide a seamless experience for service users.
■ We all take time for continuing professional development to ensure that we offer service users an up-to-date service.
■ We all strive to maintain and improve the quality of services.
■ We value our staff and morale is high.

Your list might be much longer.

The next stage is to take the list itself and ask what the opposite of each of these statements would be. It might help to ask how you could make things much, much worse than they are. For example, your new list might read:

■ We all avoid working with each other and service users have to work out how to move from one service area to another.
■ No-one has time for continuing professional development but it doesn't matter because service users like the way we offer the service.
■ We do things as we always have, so we'll maintain services and the quality is fine as it is.
■ We don't value our staff and morale is low.

When you read these two lists you will probably think that your organisation is somewhere between these extremes for each statement (unless you are horrified to find that the second list sounds very like the current situation).

The third stage is the important one if you are to develop some new ways of thinking. Take each of the statements in the second list and ask what you could do to change things to achieve a situation like those described in the first list. Try to work with each statement and look for practical achieveable steps. Make a new list for each statement. For example, the list for the first statement might read:

■ Insist that we work together.
■ Ensure that the people whose services link or are complementary work together.
■ Help service users to move from one service area to another.

These ideas might form the basis for a practical action plan. Similar approaches to the other statements will produce further ideas that might extend the action plan.

This may seem rather simple and obvious, but it can help in situations where everything seems to have complex connections that make it too difficult to take any action. Staff might also feel overworked and listless, without any ideas about how to improve the situation for themselves or for service users. Ideas that emerge from this process can often seem simple and achievable, often without needing additional funding.

Many of us find it difficult to free ourselves from the self-imposed constraints of our regular patterns of thinking. This is particularly likely to happen when we work in familiar settings with the same people and when we have developed similar ways of thinking and approaching issues. We can, however, plan to ensure that there are opportunities to challenge our own thinking or the thinking that we do in groups.

Example 3.2:   Metaphors

One way of opening up discussion about a situation or issue is to ask individuals or small groups to think of how they might describe it as a metaphor. For example, if the issue that you want to discuss is how to make better use of your team's weekly meeting, you might divide your group into three sub-groups. Each sub-group thinks of a metaphor for the weekly meeting and has to explain to the other groups why the meeting is like that metaphor. The result might be something like this:

Group 1. Our weekly meeting is like a garden. We have lots of ideas and some fall on fertile ground and grow but lots of them just wither away, perhaps because we don't feed or water them. We could be more careful about them and maybe group things together with some fences around them or low walls. We might need to sort out what grows best in the sun and what needs more shelter. Maybe we need paths from one area to another. We might need more variety and colour. Would it be good to try to attract more birds and butterflies? Perhaps we're all bored and need to dig it up and start again.

Group 2. We thought that our meeting is like an oriental rug. It is richly patterned and has lots of colour and interest, but can seem just very busy and confusing. Maybe we could turn it into a magic carpet and do wonderful things, but somehow it stays firmly on the ground and often looks a bit tired and grubby. We often sweep the dust under it.

Group 3. Our weekly meeting is like rain. We sit there getting damper and more miserable while it pours over us from above. Now and again the water helps something to grow, but mostly we just feel soaked or even drowning.

The imagery and attitudes revealed in the responses can be helpful if the group had not realised how others thought about the meetings. This can provoke discussion in itself. The ideas can be pushed a little further, however, if the whole group then take each of the metaphors and think about what you might do in each set of circumstances and how this might be applied to the weekly meeting. For example, you can do things in a garden such as make paths or build walls and fences – how might you apply that to the weekly meeting and what effect might it have? You can clean up an oriental rug and make sure that no dust is swept under the carpet. How might that be applied to a weekly meeting? What 'dust' is allowed to be hidden unchallenged? How might you respond to heavy rain? If you bring out umbrellas and raincoats, that might suggest that the participants in the weekly meeting need opportunities to be more prepared so that they can be involved in the issues without feeling overwhelmed.

Some people find it difficult to use their imaginations, particularly in settings that they consider to require formal workplace behaviour and not social situations or settings in which they might be a little playful. It often helps to create an appropriate atmosphere before trying to stimulate creative thinking. It usually helps to move out of the normal work setting if that is fairly formal, but it is not necessary to go far away. It might be helpful to use social settings in which people feel at ease, but this will depend on the relationships within a group. As with most planning, it helps to discuss the idea with those involved and seek their co-operation in identifying a suitable setting.

It can also be helpful to discuss the difficulties that many people find in taking part in creative thinking if they feel that the activities are childish and not good use of work time. The idea of 'left and right brain' thinking is now quite widely accepted. This notion offers a perspective on creative thinking that can help those uncomfortable with the activities to explain to themselves and others why they feel as they do but also to accept that there is a different dimension to be explored.

Example 3.3:   Accessing the right side of your brain

Our brains have two sides, each with different characteristics. A broad comparison is:

Left side of the brain	Right side of the brain
verbal – uses words to describe	non-verbal – no need for words
analytic – uses step-by-step reasoning	synthetic – puts things together
symbols used to represent things	concrete – relates to things as they appear
abstract – generalises	sees likenesses, uses metaphors
sequences events in time	no sense of time
rational – uses reason and facts	nonrational
digital – uses numbers to count	spatial – relates things in space
uses logic and evidence	intuitive – uses insight, patterns, feelings
ideas have linear connections	holistic, whole patterns and structures

(adapted from Edwards, 1987, p. 40)

The danger in only using one half of our brain is that we either see the world in terms of our abstract ways of describing and measuring things or we see things only in patterns of related issues. A mix of approaches would enable us to take a more perceptive view.

Most people find it easier to start thinking with one side or the other. For example, some people set out their ideas in lists and others draw diagrams. One way you can broaden your thinking is to make deliberate use of your least favourite approach. If you are a list maker, sometimes force yourself to use mindmapping approaches (see Buzan, 1974). If you prefer to start with drawings and diagrams, try to set out your ideas in logical sequences. Usually, there is something unexpected to add to your ideas when you approach them from these different perspectives.

SYSTEMS THINKING

Systems thinking is an approach to thinking that tries to keep an overview of wholeness rather than allowing thinking to focus on individual features without considering the part that these features play in a whole system. It is based on the idea of the whole being more than the sum of its parts. For example, a ward or an operating theatre might be considered as separate units but they are also part of a system that is a hospital. They may be considered as sub-systems that contribute to the wider system. These systems consist of people, buildings and equipment, but also of less tangible features including values, beliefs, ideas and behaviours.

Peter Senge identified systems thinking as one of the five disciplines necessary for a learning organisation and, by implication, for those leading initiatives in organisations that are able to be responsive to their environments. His description of systems thinking was offered as a metaphor:

A cloud masses, the sky darkens, leaves twist upward, and we know that it will rain. We also know that after the storm, the runoff will feed into groundwater miles away, and the sky will grow clear by tomorrow. All these events are distant in time and space, and yet they are all connected within the same pattern. Each has an influence on the rest, an influence that is usually hidden from view. You can only understand the system of a rainstorm by contemplating the whole, not any individual part of the pattern.

Business and other human endeavors are also systems. They, too, are bound by invisible fabrics of interrelated actions, which often take years to fully play out their effects on each other. Since we are part of that lacework ourselves, it's doubly hard to see the whole pattern of change. Instead, we tend to focus on snapshots of isolated parts of the system, and wonder why our deepest problems never seem to get solved. Systems thinking is a conceptual framework, a body of knowledge and tools that has been developed over the past fifty years, to make the full patterns clearer, and to help us see how to change them effectively.

(Senge, 1990, pp. 6–7)

In thinking about a system, we define it with a boundary that separates what we consider to be inside the system from what is outside and not part of that system. Each element that is inside the system is connected to others and is both affected by other elements and affects them too. It is this mutually dependent aspect of the elements in a system that makes it important to consider the whole whenever we consider the component parts, particularly if we are thinking about making any changes. Making a change in one component part of a system will have an effect on all other elements in that system and consequently on the whole. Thinking about the wholeness is a holistic approach.

Some key ideas about systems thinking are:

- Everything in a system is connected together – the elements are interconnected.
- A system does something, produces something, has an output. Only those elements that contribute to production of that output are valid components of a system.
- A system has a boundary and exists in an environment. For example, a hospital might be defined as a system and it exists in a social, political, economic and technological environment as well as a geographic location.
- A system is defined by your own thinking and focus. In approaching a problem or issue holistically your own focus defines the system. You can include or leave out elements that you consider do not directly relate to the focus of your interest as long as you retain an overview, a holistic view of the system, and avoid considering only one feature or issue in isolation.
- A system can have sub-systems.

Systems thinking involves taking a holistic view of a situation so that when you identify the systems within a setting you notice how they link with each other and with other elements in the setting.

The first stage in this approach to thinking is development of awareness of the whole and the parts that make up the whole. From this awareness you can engage with the elements and issues and develop a more detailed understanding of the context and the inter-action of features within it. From this detailed but contextualised understanding you can consider how to manage the situation so that the systems can work more smoothly to achieve their outcomes. Many people now talk of taking a 'whole systems approach' to any improvement or change to ensure that the overall result of any action is fully considered.

In this chapter we have considered a number of different approaches to thinking. As a leader it is important to be open to different approaches and viewpoints and it is helpful to have some understanding of different ways of thinking. If some of these approaches are very new ideas to you, you may want to follow up the references given here to gain more confidence in thinking in different ways.

CHAPTER 4

LEARNING TO CHANGE

In this chapter we pursue the idea that learning is crucial to change. We consider how learning contributes to change in health and care services. Services are essentially about interpersonal relationships and therefore the learning experiences of service providers and users are central to service development.

The first section of the chapter focuses on how we learn and develop as adults and what helps or hinders us. We then consider the experience of transformative learning, which is significant personal development. Transformative learning contributes to the ways in which we anticipate and visualise change and helps to explain some of the experiences we have during significant change.

An understanding of transformative learning is also helpful in considering what we mean by transformative leadership. Any change impacts on individuals in a variety of ways and can force them into learning and development that they are unprepared for. Leading change and transformation brings responsibilities for supporting learning.

Health and social care services are delivered in a society in which change is constant. Change means that we have to learn to think and to do things differently. For anyone working in health and care services, an ability to continue learning is essential.

LEARNING IN HEALTH AND SOCIAL CARE

Many people used to think that learning was something that children did in school and that there was no need to carry on learning once schooling was completed and academic or professional qualifications gained. This is no longer true, if it ever was, and now we all have to continue learning throughout our working lives. We are also more aware now of the difference between formal education and learning as a normal activity in life. Our formal education is intended to provide a foundation for life and work but much of our learning comes from our personal experience. Learning as continuing professional development and lifelong learning as part of living a full life are now considered to be important to everyone working in health and social care.

Peter Jarvis defines learning as 'the transformation of experience into knowledge, skills and attitudes' (Jarvis, 1987, p. 8). He goes on to note that learning takes place through a variety of processes. We have considerable choice in how we might approach learning. Many people like to engage in formal learning (education and training in structured courses) but there are also many informal ways of learning. Some like to gain an overview from books or from watching or asking others before trying things out for themselves.

Much of our work in health and care services is practical and is carried out through interpersonal contact. This raises a number of issues in terms of learning. All of our actions are informed by mental models, concepts and theories, whether these are consciously selected or unconsciously accepted. These conceptual ideas are sometimes referred to as fields of practice and study. Our actions take place in a field of practice. We learn to link ideas from the field of study to activities in the field of practice. As our work involves both theory and application in practice, both types of learning are important.

'There is increasing evidence that lifelong learning, as part of good employment practice, lies at the heart of effective organisational performance.' (Department of Health, *Working Together – Learning Together*, 2001)

One of the difficulties we face is that nothing stands still for very long, and both theory and practice are constantly changing. It is not sufficient to only continue learning about the field of study, even if that is the main area of your work, as the field of practice continually changes and evolves. Theory becomes out of date as new ideas and discoveries replace older theories. Practice also changes as new procedures and processes replace older ones in response to development in our knowledge about the impact of our actions. We also have to change and develop practice to accommodate new technology and processes.

Health and care services are no longer considered to be adequate if they operate in isolated packages, particularly when a service user has to progress from one service to another in order to receive a complete service. One of the main concerns in modernisation of public services is to provide a seamless service in which all linked services are joined up so that from the user's perspective the service is experienced as seamless. This cannot be achieved unless those providing each area of service understand each others' work. The increasing emphasis on working across professional, disciplinary and agency boundaries reflects attempts to reduce barriers that inhibit seamless service provision. Many people find that working together is easier if learning is also shared.

In services that are so personal, the service user is also a learner. As patients and clients of health and care services we learn more about ourselves and about the ways in which we live with our health and social welfare. Increasingly, patients and clients are seeking to be better informed about their own conditions and about what health and care services can offer them. Some patients and clients become as well informed or better informed about their particular condition than the professionals and clinicians who offer services to them. Learning with expert patients and clients is a new aspect of working life for many, particularly those who are not accustomed to having their knowledge or expertise challenged. Patients and other service users are also not always anxious to be offered choices or to find that they are expected to learn how to look after their own needs without constant expert assistance. Not only do those working in health and social care need to pay attention to their own learning needs but also to facilitating learning for service users. Learning is at the heart of so much of our working lives that those leading change in health and care services need to understand how to offer leadership in learning.

LEARNING AS AN ADULT

Ideally, people are able to learn from their experience and are able to avoid simply repeating bad or unsatisfactory experiences. Have you ever considered why some people learn from experience and others seem not to? Do you find that you learn best when you are challenged by a problem? Do you think that you learn differently as an adult from the ways in which you learnt as a child? One of the most obvious differences between adults and children is the difference in experience. Malcolm Knowles proposed that there are some characteristics of adult learners that make them different from children in their approach to learning. He suggested four significant differences:

- a change in self-concept, since adults need to be more self-directive;
- experience, since mature individuals accumulate an expanding reservoir of experience which becomes an exceedingly rich resource in learning;
- readiness to learn, since adults want to learn in the problem areas with which they are confronted and which they regard as relevant;
- orientation towards learning, since adults have a problem-centred orientation they are less likely to be subject-centred.

(Knowles, 1978, pp. 53–57)

Is this true of you? Test these ideas out in the following activity.

ACTIVITY 4.1

Allow 5 minutes.

Tick any of the following statements that you think apply to your approach to learning:

1. You prefer to be in control of what you learn and how
   you learn it.   ❐
2. You recognise that you can draw from your experience
   when you learn.   ❐
3. You are more interested in learning things that seem
   urgent or relevant.   ❐
4. You are more interested in learning when you are faced
   with a situation in which you want to understand better
   or behave differently.   ❐

Once we no longer have to go to school we can largely choose what
we learn for our own interest and amusement. We do, however, often
have to learn to do new things as part of our work. If you have had
formal training and also learnt 'on the job' you might be able to compare the difference between learning to a set timetable and syllabus
and learning from what happens around you and how you respond.

Those who regularly reflect on their practice will know how much
can be learnt from experience, not just from having lots of experience but from thinking about why you behaved as you did and what
other options there were that you might not have considered. Would
you do the same again in similar circumstances or would you do
something differently in order to achieve better results?

Some of us can confidently say that we are quick learners when we
want to 'get up to speed' with a new topic or issue. Some can motivate themselves and plan a way of learning that they are confident
works for them. We will consider some ways of doing that. You
might, however, have thought of times when you tried to learn something that you were not very interested in or thought that you were
not naturally 'good' at. Many people feel that they are no good at
mathematics because they did badly at school, but most of these people manage their money well enough and can add up purchases in a
shop. Others say that they are no good at art or music and may be
missing potentially fulfilling aspects of life. It is helpful to be aware
of messages that we received when we were children and to remember that these are not necessarily messages that help us as adults.

As an adult learning you will probably:

- think independently;
- value experience;
- make judgements;
- analyse against experience;
- decide your own priorities;
- set your own targets;
- work out your own strategies;
- make up your own mind.

Knowles suggested that as an adult learning you will want to draw from your own experience and to be able to apply what you are learning in current problem areas. Another obvious aspect of being an adult is that you are older than a child. Age brings experience but there is more involved if you are to learn from that experience and not just repeat similar experiences over and over again.

Learning in practical situations may bring opportunities to learn alongside experts who can show you approaches that generally work. However, in some situations there are few experts to ask. These situations are more like those you encounter when trying to learn a new language or when you are developing relationships with other people. You depend on feedback to assess your progress and you cannot receive feedback until you have taken some action. Learning from experience is heavily reliant on making use of feedback. If you are unfamiliar with this, you may need to develop skills in collecting and using feedback.

Another aspect of learning from experience is that people learn in different ways. As individuals are all different, there are differences in the things that help or hinder our learning.

ACTIVITY 4.2

Allow 10 minutes.

Consider some of your own recent learning experiences. Try to think of something that you learnt that involved both theory and application of the ideas in practice. Ask yourself what helps you to learn and what hinders your learning.

Make a list under each heading:

Things that help me to learn   Things that hinder my learning

_____   _____
_____   _____
_____   _____
_____   _____
_____   _____
_____   _____

Do your lists show positive and negative sides of learning? For example, you might say that it helps you to learn if you can have lots of time, but you might know yourself well enough to know that you need deadlines to get round to doing things. Did you say that motivation helps you to learn? The other side of wanting to learn very much is that too much pressure to succeed can freeze you into being unable to do anything. Did you list encouragement as something that helps? However, sometimes this can seem like interference and too much pressure to achieve something that someone else wants you to do. As in most aspects of life, balance is important in learning!

Some of the other barriers to learning that people have identified include prejudice and hostility from peers, unfamiliar use of language and jargon (although managers usually want to understand the jargon of management), difficulties in concentration, feeling patronised, feeling lack of confidence and feeling unprepared. Some people may have little support from their families or from work colleagues. Also, of course, some people have disabilities that may have to be overcome in different ways.

Some of the things which encourage people to learn include support and encouragement, feedback that learning is successful, opportunities to try out new ways of doing things, resources to pay for and to give time for learning and other people to show interest in your learning. For some people it is important to have a strong personal reason for engaging in learning. However, for others it may seem too mechanistic to set formal objectives and be more helpful to identify wide and open goals.

Another aspect of learning is that the personal process of learning takes place in a context, it is not isolated from the world in which we live. Much of our learning is stimulated by noticing something that seems not to 'fit' into the understanding that we thought we had about the world around us. We discuss our ideas with other people. The feedback we receive about our ideas and actions comes from other people. Learning is a social activity:

> People are a result of learning and continue to be what they are because of learning. Whilst learning and living are not the same phenomenon, they are co-terminus and those who help others learn (whether or not they are called teachers) bear some of the responsibility for helping people grow and develop through the complexities of social life, but that is a human responsibility since people are and must be interdependent because they live in societies.
>
> (Jarvis, 1987, p. 206)

Jarvis associates learning with growing and developing in complex social settings. He suggests that we are, to some extent, socialised into the culture of the setting we inhabit, the knowledge, values, beliefs and attitudes of those around us. We may not even be aware of this until we find ourselves in an unfamiliar culture when some of our beliefs, values or assumptions are challenged. In health and social care services we experience many different cultures. There is the cultural richness of colleagues and service users who come from different social and religious backgrounds, the cultures that have developed among many professional and clinical staff (particularly those who have shared formal education to achieve registration) and there are cultures that develop within agencies and organisations. When we recognise a different perspective brought by someone who holds a different view of the world from the one we have formed we often find our own viewpoint challenged. This can lead to a profound learning experience in which we review the assumptions and beliefs that we have relied on as a personal 'frame of reference' and realise that some of these fundamental values are outdated or inappropriate for the lives we now live. Learning that leads to a fundamental change of view is called transformative learning.

TRANSFORMATIVE LEARNING

Jack Mezirow suggested that age brings an ability to view life from a wider perspective:

> to the degree our culture permits, we tend to move through adulthood along a maturity gradient which involves a sequential restructuring of one's frame of reference for making and under-standing meanings. We move through successive transformations towards analysing things from a perspective increasingly removed from one's personal or local perspective.
>
> (cited in Jarvis, 1987, p. 18)

Are you aware of having changed your view at different times, perhaps as a result of moving into a new role or situation? Were you able then to look back and see things differently? You may have changed the way you see or understand something because of being confronted with a new idea or attitude.

One of the difficulties many people face when they take on a new role in a familiar workplace setting is that the role puts them into a different position and they are expected to take a different viewpoint. Although you may continue to do some of the work that you did before, your responsibilities are different, perhaps wider. You may become the person who is expected to support and help others, perhaps to supervise their work and to take responsibility for comple-tion of tasks. People moving into management roles are often aware of this sort of change in their frame of reference as they begin to see the activities of their organisation from a different perspective. From a management perspective you may find that there is more to under-stand although you may not find it easy to see the 'bigger picture'.

Learning in the workplace involves many different types of learning because your thoughts and ideas influence your actions and the ways in which you interact with other people. Transformative learning can change more than the way in which you work, it can change the way in which you live your life – consider the different development stages suggested in Example 4.1.

Example 4.1:   Stages of personal development

Perry (in Cross, 1981, p. 180) developed a hierarchy of developmental stages explicitly related to perceptions of education linked to intellectual and ethical development. Perry proposed that we go through nine stages of development:

- At the first stage a learner sees the world in right/wrong terms and expects an ultimate authority, often a teacher, to tell them what is right.
- At the second stage, when there is uncertainty, or difference of opinion, the authority might be thought to be at fault or might be blamed for forcing learners to find out for themselves.
- At the third stage the learner accepts that diversity and uncertainty are legitimate, but believes that this is a temporary situation because authorities have not yet found the right answer.
- By the fourth stage the learner perceives that uncertainty and diversity of opinion are legitimate but suspects that they are associated with what different ultimate authorities want.
- At the fifth stage the learner recognises that all knowledge and values, including those of any authority, exist in relationship to their contexts. They also realise that notions of right and wrong are also subject to the conditions in any particular context.
- The understanding gained in the fifth stage leads to the realisation that individuals have to find their own orientations in a world in which everything is relative. This is much more difficult than committing themselves to a belief in certainty and absolute authority.
- At the seventh stage the learner makes an initial commitment to some values and beliefs.
- From this position, the learner experiences the implications of making this commitment and discovers the responsibilities it brings.
- The final ninth stage entails the development of identity among the multiple responsibilities associated with commitment. The learner realises that commitment is an ongoing, unfolding activity through which people express themselves and their life-styles.

The way in which we react to change is affected by our stage of development. Some may comply unquestioningly with orders from an authority (as in the first and second stage). Others will be unwilling but comply because they accept the authority and expect it to always be right. Others will have reached the fifth stage and may question what is right if situations and contexts change. Those who review their own assumptions, values and beliefs may find that they need to make some personal changes and adopt different commitments. This brings changes in identity that can have profound implications for individuals.

PLANNING YOUR OWN LEARNING

One aspect of leadership involves taking responsibility for yourself. If you are convinced that learning is important to growth, development and change, you will want to consider your own attitudes and approaches to learning. Megginson and Pedler outline steps for a development route for managers:

- personal desire to learn – some dissatisfaction or discomfort with the present state;
- self-diagnosis – understanding of why you need to change;
- setting goals for self-development, ideally measurable ones;
- take a risk – this is the shift from current state to new state and builds confidence;
- design a programme to support you to reach the goals;
- recognise the contribution friends and colleagues can make in encouraging and giving feedback;
- keep on with the programme – stickability and perseverance;
- assess yourself against the goals, leading to satisfaction and confidence in using the process again or dissatisfaction and a return to the beginning of the process.

(Megginson and Pedler, 1992, pp. 4–7)

We may not recognise our own incompetence until we see a competent performance and realise that we are not yet competent. Later we may be able to perform so easily that we become unaware of our level of competence. We progress through a sequence of being:

- unconsciously incompetent
- consciously incompetent
- consciously competent
- unconsciously competent.

These steps can apply equally well to anyone wanting to make their own plan for learning. You can start by identifying an area in which you want to learn more and clarifying what you think needs to change. For example, you may feel that you do not understand enough about the environment in which your agency or organisation works. This may be because you only see the service users who come into your area of service and you often feel frustrated that other services do not seem to be as efficient or helpful as they might be to complement what you are trying to do. The frustration you feel may be the trigger to find out more and to try to understand why the overall service is not as good as you would like it to be.

Once you have identified the area of learning and clarified why it is important for you, you can think about how you might set a target for this learning. It is important to set a target because if you don't, how will you know whether you have learnt what you intend? But a target for learning has to be stated in a way that focuses on the purpose. It can help to start with 'I will be able to . . .' and complete the sentence with one of the things that you want to be able to do differently. For example, you might state, 'I will be able to describe and explain the importance of the key factors in our environment that impact on our service provision.' That will help you to understand, but will not be enough to reduce your frustration with inadequate service provision. You might add, 'I will be able to identify potential areas for service improvement.' In any service improvement there will be a number of other people, staff and service users, who will also need to do things a little differently if anything is changed. If you are to make a difference you will need to agree the nature of the change with them and gain their support. You might add this as a learning outcome – 'I will be able to identify and communicate effectively with the key people whose co-operation will be needed to make service improvements.' Of course, this does not yet lead you to taking action, so you might add, 'I will be able to develop agreement about what to do to improve our service and secure support to enable us to carry out the improvement.' You will only be able to review the full sequence of these learning objectives when you have reached the point at which you can move into implementing a change. At that stage you may want to make a new learning plan to deal with all the issues that arise in implementing change.

Learning outcomes that involve understanding, discussion and negotiation cannot be achieved by only reading a book or taking a course. You will need to gain experience and seek feedback on your performance if you are to evaluate your developing abilities. You will need to create opportunities to encourage others to question and challenge your ideas if you are to understand the different perspectives that might be held on what you propose as an improvement. How will you do this?

Many people find that the most effective programmes of learning are created from mixtures of approaches, blended to suit the environment and the focus that you have taken. For example, you might consider shadowing some of the senior managers, clinicians and professionals in the organisations and agencies that contribute to the range of services in which your area of work lies to gain more understanding of the day-to-day issues that impact on service provision. Alongside this, you might consult your organisation's business plan and strategic plan to understand what your organisation plans to do with the resources at its disposal. Any proposal for improvement is unlikely to gain support unless it can demonstrate that it will contribute to achieving the overall strategic objectives. You will also need to create opportunities to learn more about how the different elements in your services interact with each other. There are many ways that you might approach that area of learning. You might examine the organisational charts and enquire whether there are any diagrams of how one area of service links with another. You might identify key individuals and make appointments to interview them about the links they make and how they review the effectiveness of service continuity. You might follow a number of service users through their use of linked services or ask them about their experiences.

As you can see, learning plans can become quite complicated and it can require quite long periods of time to achieve outcomes of this nature. You can reduce the complexity by focusing on something that would contribute to this longer-term aim. For example, you might set yourself only the first learning outcome to start with, so that you could feel confident in pursuing further ones once you had gained some success.

Most learners need support from others to pursue learning plans. You might consider enlisting the support of one or more of your colleagues, perhaps agreeing to help each other to achieve objectives. If your learning is to link closely with your day-to-day work you will probably want to involve your line manager, who would be able to offer practical support if you need to adapt your working schedules to shadow or talk to people in other parts of the service. Many people would also find the involvement of someone from their training or human resources department helpful both in supporting their plans and in helping to make useful contacts. Many also find it very helpful to have a mentor to act as both support and challenge and to help to keep things in perspective. If your learning plan involves learning about how to take a role that you have not previously taken, you might be able to secure support to shadow someone in that role or even to 'act up' in a more senior role for a period to gain appropriate experience.

Example 4.2:   Action learning

Many people find it helpful to have a regular forum in which to discuss their own progress and the barriers that they face personally in progressing their learning or projects. Action learning sets are often used to provide a forum in which these discussions can take place. Each individual is both supported and challenged and offers both support and challenge to the other set members. It is usual for each set member to bring a project that might be a formal workplace project or it might be an area of development that will be approached in a variety of different ways. Most sets agree action points for each individual that are reviewed at the next set meeting and many find this discipline useful. Normally it is helpful for a learning set to have a facilitator when it forms to help the set to develop working patterns and focal areas for each individual. Once members become confident and experienced in contributing to action learning it may not be necessary to have a facilitator. Action learning is often very successful in helping individuals to gain insights into their learning and work:

> When I first came across the concept of action learning I had a degree of cynicism and hesitation. As both a participant in action learning sets and as an observer of the value of the process to others, I now believe the concentration on and support for the learning of the individual results in a speed and depth of learning and often 'cognitive leaps' which other processes do not engender.
>
> (Jon Bareham quoted in McGill and Beaty, 1992)

(You can read more about Action learning in McGill and Beaty 1992).

Your plans might also include linking learning from experience with formal courses that can lead to qualifications. Many academic courses now include emphasis on applying theoretical ideas to practical situations and you are often able to carry out projects as vehicles for learning and to gain qualifications from assessment of the learning that you have gained from the process of investigation and implementation. Critical reflective practice is now expected in most professional education and it provides an approach that can be used subsequently for continuing professional development (CPD) throughout your career.

LEADING TRANSFORMATIVE LEARNING

Once you consider the implications of transformative learning for individuals, you can appreciate why it is often so difficult for people to engage with and accept change. Most of us accept that we have to learn and develop throughout our lives and that incidents we experience will often provoke such learning and development. Often these incidents puzzle us or cause emotional reactions such as anger, fear or frustration. We may feel that we will lose something that we value or that we will face difficult challenges in the proposed new conditions. We often find that our ideas and our values are challenged and we have to re-think our priorities and reconsider our value framework. These are uncomfortable things to do. People often say that learning should be fun, but transformative learning is rarely fun because it affects us so deeply although it may ultimately be very satisfactory and rewarding.

In this chapter we have considered the part that learning plays in change. Leading change involves leading transformation and to achieve this any individuals involved have to engage to some degree in transformative learning. As a leader, you have a responsibility to recognise that each person will respond in a different way as they face the challenges to their current ways of thinking and acting. Although some individuals will welcome an opportunity to learn and develop, some will be neither willing nor emotionally prepared. Leading change and transformation brings the opportunity to share learning and development in a context that delivers benefits to service users and staff. It also brings responsibilities for supporting learning.

CHAPTER 5

TAKING A LEADING ROLE

This chapter is about some of the issues that you might face in taking on a leadership role and ways in which you might prepare yourself. For those with leadership experience, we also discuss continuing development as a leader. The chapter begins by looking at how a person becomes a leader and what the role entails. We then explore the competence and skills that a leader needs in a health and social care setting. We also consider how you might react when you become a leader, how you might prepare and how you can take care of yourself as a leader.

OPPORTUNITIES TO LEAD

How do people become leaders? Health and social care services are full of people who are leading different initiatives and projects. How has this happened?

ACTIVITY 5.1

Allow 5 minutes.

How do people become leaders? Think about leaders that you know in different areas of work. Make a note of four ways that a person can become a leader.

1 _____
2 _____
3 _____
4 _____

Perhaps the most obvious way for people to become leaders is to be appointed to a leadership role. This might happen if someone is asked to 'lead up this project' or to 'take a lead in getting this started' or, more formally, to 'head up' a new initiative. This often happens when an organisation sets goals that can be progressed through projects that require leaders. For example, when two organisations agree to collaborate more closely to deliver more integrated services, each of the service areas involved might be treated as a separate project, each with a project leader and team.

Sometimes a person attains a leadership position because she or he has a personal interest in an initiative. An individual with the enthusiasm to make progress with an idea might gain support from others to take the development forward. A leader is often the person who cares most about getting something done and so willingly takes on the responsibility to enthuse others. An example of this type of leader might often be found in a clinical or professional area where one individual leads in introducing a new way of working that offers improved benefits to patients or clients.

Another way that someone might become a leader is when there is a vacuum in an area of activity and this person finds that they are concerned and able enough to encourage others to move forward. Leadership of this type might arise when one area of service provision is less effective than other services that depend on it for their own service delivery. For example, if transport services for patients travelling to a clinic are unreliable, patients will often be late for appointments or miss them altogether. A clinician might take on the lead responsibility of developing better relationships with those who provide the transport in order to improve the links between these services.

You might have also thought of a leader who was not very willing but whom others encouraged to take a lead because the person was thought to be right for the job. For example, a junior secretary who had a popular idea about how to improve a record form might be asked by colleagues to take a lead in testing out the idea. This might include drafting a proposal for improvement and gathering feedback about whether the proposal would meet the needs of all those who had to use the form.

There are many different ways in which a person might become a leader.

You might have noticed that the examples of how someone might become a leader all have implications of leading some sort of progression or change. Leading is a word that implies movement, direction and purpose and these are aspects of leadership that you can learn to develop. Leadership is not only about having personal skills, it is also about attitudes, commitment, ability to attract support and less tangible qualities including vision and integrity. Let us look at these more closely.

BECOMING A COMPETENT LEADER

People in health and social care are generally familiar with the notion of competence. Competence includes more than we might mean by a skill because it also encompasses the knowledge that underpins a skilled performance and the attitudes that ensure that the performance is appropriate in its context.

For the first time in 2001 the National Health Service in England identified a set of core skills that any worker in health services would be expected to be able to demonstrate ('Working Together – Learning Together. A framework for the Lifelong Learning for the NHS'). This measure was taken to provide a systematic framework for development to support the overall strategy of modernising services. Lifelong learning was recognised as being at the heart of effective organisational performance and the strategy was designed to equip staff to:

- support changes and improvement in patient care;
- take advantage of wider career opportunities;
- realise their potential.

The strategy was designed to support staff in a context in which everyone would experience changing patterns of healthcare delivery and increasing expectations of work and learning. There was an emphasis on equal opportunities and recognition of increasing diversity in society and also recognition of the implications of policy commitments to increase the use of new technology.

The core skills identified as being necessary for all staff, regardless of their role or level in health services, were:

- respecting the rights and feelings of patients and families;
- communicating effectively with patients and colleagues;
- using information effectively and sensitively;
- understanding how the NHS and their local organisation work;
- working effectively in teams;
- keeping skills and competence up to date;
- contributing to health and safety.

This is a useful list to start with when considering the competencies that any leader needs in health and care services.

Respect for others is essential for development of inclusive and democratic processes. Without respect we cannot participate in team-working or listen attentively to colleagues or service users. We also cannot respect rights if we don't know what they are. You might like to think about what you consider to be basic human rights – those that you expect to experience yourself. Another area of rights are those that are rights by law. Your area of work may be subject to many different legal requirements – there will certainly be legal frameworks governing the employment of staff, health and safety and management of confidential information. There may well also be legislation governing how you work with service users, for example the laws relating to responsibility for children.

Communication is another core competence that most of us need to continue to develop throughout our working lives. Consider how closely and attentively you listen and whether you are able to encourage others to communicate with you. You are probably a very busy person, so how do you make yourself available for communication with others when your time is so precious? Are you aware of being a better communicator in face-to-face settings than you are when using a phone or e-mail? Do you write clearly and without unintentionally causing offence? Do you ever get involved in muddles because of poor communications? These are things to think about when you are considering your own potential areas for development.

Information handling is another area of competence that demands a mixture of knowledge and skills. Do you know your responsibilities under the most recent data protection act and is confidential information kept appropriately in your area of work? Local policies often detail agreed procedures. Do you know what management information systems are used by your organisation? If you take a role in leading an initiative you will often need to access up-to-date information as quickly as possible. Again, you will probably be able to identify some personal development areas related to use of information.

It is difficult for anyone now to keep up with developments in health and care services. Many staff in health and social care know little about how their own organisation or area of service works. Now that much of the restructuring is intended to improve the links between services, it has become more important to know how your area of work connects to others. The service user experience of services often identifies gaps that those who work in services are less likely to notice. We usually have to make a deliberate effort to find out more about the areas of work that we do not deal with in our day-to-day work. Again, you will probably be able to identify some learning and development needs for yourself in this area of competence.

Teamworking is one of the basic areas of competence and the setting in which leadership is particularly evident. Teams often change and new teams are formed to work on projects, so competence in identifying learning and development needs, making and implementing plans and reviewing development is important. Also, team development has some different dynamics and it is helpful if all team members have some understanding of how teams work. As we discussed in Chapter 2, leaders and teamworkers are a collective in which roles may frequently change.

The last two of the core competencies, keeping up to date and taking responsibility for health and safety, can also be considered as potential development areas for everyone, regardless of the stage in your career or how much you have learnt about these areas in the past.

There are, however, many other skills and competencies that are also relevant for leaders. It is widely accepted that leaders need to be able to build a vision with others and inspire them to want to work towards achieving the future that they can imagine together. Once there is a shared vision, leaders are those who develop a shared sense of direction and purpose to enable progress towards achievement of the vision. There will be many different perspectives and potential conflict, so negotiation skills will often be needed. It is difficult to maintain clarity about the direction and purpose unless the under-pinning principles and values have been thoroughly discussed and agreed. When there are disagreements and anxieties, the integrity of the leader will be questioned and the leader's own values and concerns will often be challenged. It is very helpful for a leader to demonstrate passion and commitment, but there will be people who want to assure themselves that these are real and not just acted in an attempt to motivate others. So leaders have to be very aware of their own motivations and the ways in which they derive their own commitment from this. The attitudes of leaders are always under some degree of scrutiny and will influence the extent to which they are able to attract support.

'Painful moments are good times to learn. . . . The focus of our energy on others needs to be redirected to ourselves. Instead of "why did she behave so aggressively?" I should be asking: "What was it about her aggressive behaviour that triggered something in me?"' (April, Macdonald and Vriesendorp, 2000, p. 9)

Awareness is essential for leaders in health and social care. Not only are the services complex and often sensitive, but service users depend on consistent service provision. We need to be aware of the wider implications of anything we do, so awareness is an important quality to develop. Awareness includes noticing issues and develop-ments, being sensitive to the undercurrents as well as the open and easily accessed information and interpretations. If you are aware, you will have noticed and taken an interest in the issues that are taking peoples' attention and you will also have thought about the impli-cations for those people and for their work. Awareness involves being able to collect and interpret a variety of different sorts of data and being able to make connections between what you understand to be happening and the implications for your area of work. Awareness is not only the usual starting point for alerting others to the need to change, but also essential during a change process to ensure that everything progresses in the agreed direction.

Another important area of competence for a leader is an ability to work across traditional boundaries. There are many boundaries in health and social care, both formal and informal. The formal bound-aries include those between organisations and agencies, but we increasingly need to work more closely with those in other structures to reduce the gaps in services. We also often need to work across the boundaries that have grown between professions and also those that have developed between some areas of practice. With the development of more flexible working it has become easier to work and learn alongside people from different areas of services and you might consider extending your experience if it is currently rather limited. Personal flexibility is important in a leader and you might consider whether you have stretched your own limits recently.

One more area of competence frequently mentioned in connection with leadership is the ability to develop a personal network of contacts. This ability comes naturally to some but not to others, who often do not understand why it is important. Networking is important because it enables you to form social contact with people from areas of work outside your own. You know how much information and discussion is shared within a working group and how it contributes to the awareness and understanding of all of those in the group. Networking is a way of accessing some of that experience with people from backgrounds and areas of work different from your own. It can help significantly in keeping your knowledge and understanding of service development up to date, it can offer insights into the benefits and constraints experienced in different areas of work and it can help you to develop a broader perspective on your own area of work.

BEING EFFECTIVE

You need to be effective to be able to contribute as a leader. Effectiveness is about doing the right things – this implies a number of abilities. Being effective includes being able to:

- investigate and agree with others what are the right things to do in a particular situation;
- attract enough support and enthusiasm for action so that the ideas can be implemented;
- maintain momentum until objectives are achieved;
- review and revise activities to ensure that the desired outcomes are being achieved.

In most change situations, effectiveness requires a mixture of leadership commitment and management of activities. Effectiveness does not come just from learning a few skills and techniques. Skills and techniques are important and necessary, but effectiveness is more complex than that. It depends on you, the job you do, the people you work with, the other resources you have at your disposal, the organisation you work in, and the wider world with which your organisation must interact. You may need to develop your awareness of how these factors can affect your work.

ACTIVITY 5.2

Allow 15 minutes.

This activity will help you to identify some of the factors upon which effectiveness depends. You may find your answers to the questions helpful in identifying personal areas for development.

Think about a piece of work you recently carried out. This might have been an improvement in your area of work or an occasional, but more routine, activity. Choose something that was fairly complex, something that you had to think about and plan to some extent and something that involved other people. Answer the following questions about the activity. (If you prefer, you could apply this exercise to a project or major objective that you are just about to start work on: e.g. to what extent will the outcome be influenced?)

Did you feel adequately prepared to take on the task?

Did you have a clear understanding of what was required?

To what extent was the outcome influenced by your own level of competence?

Did you bring particular skills or knowledge to the situation?

To what extent were your actions influenced by personal or professional values?

What contribution did others make to the outcome, positively or negatively?

How critical were the abilities and attitudes that others brought to the situation?

Did you have the influence in your organisation that was required to achieve the task?

Do you feel that your role allows all your abilities to be brought into play?

Does it make demands that you feel unable to respond to?

All of these questions refer to aspects of work that you can think about before taking action. Preparation for a complex task can be, to some extent, a rehearsal for the real thing. If you start a major task by considering what is involved and what you are trying to achieve, this will clarify the direction and purpose of your work. If others are to be involved in achieving the outcome, you will need to develop a shared understanding of direction and purpose. It is then possible to consider how the desired outcomes will be achieved – what steps are needed to achieve each of the outcomes. This is the planning stage.

Once these steps are expressed as separate tasks, you have created an agenda for action. You can then think, probably as a group, about who should carry out each of the tasks. Your planning at this stage will include consideration of who has the necessary skills and experience or who could be supported to develop the necessary skills with appropriate supervision. In health and social care settings you will also have to consider who has the appropriate professional or clinical background and qualifications for some of the activities, and this may raise the question of your ability to bring people from different backgrounds together to work effectively. You might also need to have sufficient influence in your organisation to secure other necessary resources. All of this may seem daunting, but much of your effectiveness as a leader will result from your management ability to plan and co-ordinate the work of other people. Once you have reached the stage of carrying out activities, there is still a further stage of review. This is crucial in making sure that your actions are leading in the direction you intended.

The simple sequence of 'plan, do, review' is a useful way to remember these stages.

If you have set clear objectives it is relatively easy to review progress to establish whether these are being achieved. Reviewing progress is not simply a matter of indicating your perception of how things are going. You must also give careful consideration to other people's views about what has been done and what needs to be done (which may mean the perceptions of service users, your team and other colleagues, your manager and other managers, people in collaborating organisations).

TAKING CARE OF YOURSELF AS A LEADER

The transition into a leadership role takes place over a period of time as new challenges are encountered. Some people find that, in taking on a leadership role, they are expected to give up the specialist roles that they have performed well and with satisfaction in the past, and they may be reluctant to do this. Others – particularly in health and social care – find that they are expected to retain some of their former specialist or professional functions while taking on a leadership role as well, and finding an appropriate balance between these is not always easy. It is a tension that has to be managed.

The second aspect is the transition process itself. Here the problems highlighted are typical of those encountered by anyone moving into a new job, and not simply those of someone moving into a leading role. They are also likely to be encountered by your colleagues when they take up new positions. As a leader and team-worker you will need to be sensitive to the problems others face in adjusting to new and different demands. You may also encounter similar transitions yourself in the future when you are required to work in a different way, perhaps with colleagues to achieve a more integrated service or perhaps to move on to more responsible appointments. An understanding of the process of transition will stand you in good stead.

You may be required to provide professional leadership as well as leadership in initiating an organisational change. You may face conflicts between different values and competing priorities. It is important to be clear about what you should and should not do, and why. There will be occasions when only you have the professional skill to do a particular task, or when you are the only one with sufficient knowledge and experience to make a professional judgement or to take a particular decision. However, there will be occasions when it will make more sense to delegate certain tasks to suitably qualified members of your team, reserving yourself for tasks that others simply cannot do. There will also be occasions when you will want to encourage others to do tasks (under appropriate supervision) that will help members of your team to develop their professional skills. You may be in a small team where you have to take a regular turn in direct service provision. There is always a tension in managing these dual roles.

Example 5.1:   Self-esteem and the transition process

Some helpful research was done in this area (Adams, Hayes and Hopson, 1976). It deals with transitions in general, rather than being exclusively concerned with roles at work, but a fairly common pattern emerges for all transitions.

These researchers identified seven phases that can be predicted in a transition, from the start of the change to the point at which the change has been accepted:

1   *Immobile* – In this initial state many people feel frozen; unable to understand or to make plans. This might be because the change involves something very unfamiliar. The expectations raised may also overwhelming. If the

transition is welcome, for example a promotion or a welcome responsibility, the positive feelings may reduce the feeling of immobilisation.

2   *Minimising* – One way of getting out of this immobilisation, essentially, is by minimising the change or disruption. Very often, people will deny that the change even exists. Denial can be a reaction to a crisis too overwhelming to face head-on. In health and social care we might recognise this in ourselves or in our colleagues when we face changes that are almost too big to comprehend. Often, too, people project euphoric feelings.

3   *Depression* – Once people become aware of the reality of the change they begin to get depressed, even if they made the change voluntarily. This dip in feelings may be because of frustration because of the new demands that must be met or a feeling of not being able to cope with the new situation. Some people feel incompetent if they have to learn to do new things, particularly if they used to be very good at their previous job. People at this stage often feel angry and may blame others. There may be a sense of panic and a feeling of things disintegrating and getting out of control. This is usually when people feel most uncomfortable.

4   *Accepting* – This marks something of a turning point, as the previous stages have demonstrated some degree of holding on to the past. Movement into this stage involves 'letting go' of the past situations and accepting the new reality, saying 'Okay, here I am now; here is what I have; here's what I want'. As this is accepted as the new reality, the person's feelings begin to rise once more. They can become more optimistic about the future.

5   *Testing* – The person becomes much more active and starts *testing* himself or herself in relation to the new situation: trying out new behaviours, new life-styles, and new ways of coping with the transition. There is a tendency also at this point for people to stereotype, to have categories and classifications of the ways things and people should or should not be relative to the new situation. A lot of personal energy is available during this phase and, as they begin to deal with the new reality, it is not unlikely that those in transition will easily become frustrated and irritable.

6   *Seeking meanings* – After this burst of activity and self-testing there is a gradual shift towards wanting to understand why and how things are different – to seek meanings. This is a more conceptual activity, thinking more than acting, standing back to try to understand the meaning of the change in their lives.

7   *Internalising* – Once the change has been accepted and understood, this last stage involves incorporating the change fully into the person's life. This stage is about integration and satisfaction in the new situation.

Overall, these seven transition phases represent a cycle of experiencing disruption, gradually acknowledging its reality, testing oneself, understanding oneself, and incorporating changes in one's behaviour. The level of one's self-esteem varies across these phases and appears to follow a predictable path. Identifying the seven phases along such a self-esteem curve often gives one a better understanding of the nature of the transition cycle. This is done in Figure 5.1.

People are unlikely to move continuously from phase to phase as it has been described and diagrammed here. Any given individual's progressions and regressions are unique to his or her unique circumstances. For example, one person may never get beyond denial and minimising. Another may drop out during depression. Yet another might experience a major failure just as things begin to look up, and revert to an earlier stage in the cycle.

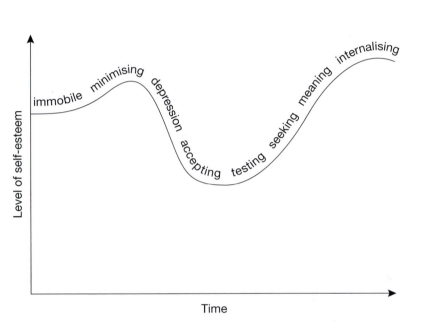

Figure 5.1   Self-esteem changes during a transition

If you are new to your role as a leader you may recognise where you are in these stages. Or you may be an experienced leader facing a transition into taking new challenging roles in a multi-disciplinary team. If you are still hanging onto the past in some way, this could be causing difficulties in managing your time and could create feelings of inadequacy if you cannot continue to deliver in all of your former roles as well as your new ones.

COPING WITH PRESSURE

Most people would agree that a certain amount of pressure is necessary to provoke action. A lot of us feel that we are at our best when the adrenaline is flowing and when we are working under pressure to achieve good results within a limited time. The problems start to arise when the pressure becomes too great or continues unabated for long periods. It then becomes stress. It ceases to be enjoyable. It becomes detrimental, even dangerous, and it can impair your effectiveness.

Stress is commonly described as a physical and psychological reaction to external forces or 'stressors'. Cranwell-Ward described stress as 'the result of an imbalance between the level of demand placed on people, as they perceive it, and their perceived capability to meet the demands' (1990, p. 8). The psychological reaction to a perceived imbalance leads to a physical reaction and the engagement of 'fight' or 'flight' mechanisms which prepare the body for action. If the cycle of stress is intermittent then the body has a chance to recover, but if the cycle becomes constantly engaged the body can suffer physical damage.

Different people, of course, react in different ways. Pressure merges into stress, almost imperceptibly. The important thing is to be able to distinguish between them, so that we can avoid stress while making the best use of pressure. The medical effects of stress are well known and include ulcers, high blood pressure, heart disease, strokes and early death. There are personal consequences and families also suffer. We need to be able to recognise stress and some of the causes of stress, and consider ways of alleviating stress.

RECOGNISING STRESS

A simple way to differentiate between pressure and stress is to think of pressure as something that comes from outside yourself and stress as the response you have when you are subjected to too much pressure. Most high achievers (and a lot of leaders would come into this category) find a degree of pressure positively motivating. They are able to respond to it energetically. Stress, on the other hand, does not produce a positive, energetic response. It is debilitating. It deprives people of their strength, their vitality and their judgement. Its effects are negative. Between these two extremes is a large inter-mediate area in which pressure merges into stress, and this is the danger area. This is where one needs constantly to be on the look-out for tell-tale signs.

Some of the more obvious signs of stress are irritability and short temper, panic reactions, heavy reliance on tobacco, alcohol or other drugs such as tranquilisers, over-busyness, insecurity, an unwilling-ness to delegate. People may become difficult to talk to, morose, confused, unable to relax, insomniac. These can all be signs of other problems, but their presence should make one suspect stress, and should suggest the need to find relief before stress leads to more damaging effects for the individual and the organisation.

CAUSES OF STRESS

The effects of stress are so serious that it is worth spending a little time considering the causes. Responsibility for the work of others is often stressful, particularly if this includes working across boundaries and integrating different areas of work. Innovation is also stressful. The social context of teamworking may bring difficulties in relationships and emotional sensitivity. Many find it stressful to be required to work more flexibly. Some aspects of roles are stressful and this can be particularly true of leadership roles when the requirements are often not very specific. There will probably be a degree of ambiguity and conflict within the roles an individual holds. There may also be overload, but even underload brings stress. Any situation with inadequate resources brings stress if you try to progress without the resources you need, and lack of control over work brings considerable stress.

ALLEVIATING STRESS

We can do many things to help to reduce stress levels in ourselves and in colleagues. We can also make our line managers and organisations aware of the problem, if it develops, and seek help.

Consider the extent to which you put pressure on yourself. As children, many of us received messages that encouraged us to try harder and to strive to do well. It is easy to continue to measure yourself by these simple childhood messages and not to reappraise the standards that you can reasonably expect of yourself as a busy adult. If you know that you put pressure on yourself to keep up a high standard in all aspects of your activities, consider whether this is causing unhelpful stress and whether there are some areas in which you could reduce the pressure.

When we experience pressure that is not excessive, we are left feeling *in control*: we know that occasionally through extra effort we can meet difficult deadlines. When pressure is excessive and we feel under stress, there is a feeling of having *lost control*: there is too much to deal with, it is too complex, we cannot see our way clear to the goal, or we are not even sure what the goal is.

As a leader you can influence the extent to which people in your setting accept stress as a way of life. In some organisations there is a tendency to take pride in working very long hours, to be seen to be at your desk very early and very late. If this is normal, people may expect to have a tense and anxious working environment and not to be able to celebrate the things that are successfully accomplished because there is always more to be done. If this sounds familiar, you can try to influence your colleagues and your team to make better use of their time and reduce the pressures put on each other.

'People who learn to master more volatile career paths also usually become more comfortable with change generally and . . . are in a better position to help their employers advance the transformation process so as to significantly improve meaningful results while minimizing the painful effects of change.'
(Kotter, 1996, p. 183)

Sometimes we feel that the work to be done simply will not fit into the time available, and this can put us under considerable stress. Revising how you use the time available can sometimes reduce this stress. You may need to identify some ways of using your time more effectively. Everyone has the same amount of time – twenty-four hours each day – but many of us feel that there is not enough time to do all the things that we want to do and all the things that we feel we have to do. There are many ways of improving your personal time management and if you feel that you need to develop your strategies this is a good area to build into your plans for self-development.

EMOTIONAL INTELLIGENCE

Emotions often run high in health and social care, where patients and carers often feel frightened and vulnerable. Many people feel angry or frustrated at being unable to heal or comfort. Anyone working in a health and care setting has to deal in some way with both their own emotional reactions and the emotional reactions of others. Goleman (1996) offered a helpful study of emotions and ways in which we might learn to live intelligently with our emotions. He proposed development of competence in self-awareness, self-control, empathy, listening, conflict resolution and co-operation. As leadership often involves being passionate and demonstrating both anger or frustration and passion about making a difference, leaders are particularly in need of this range of competencies.

Self-awareness heightens our understanding of how our own communications and behaviours impact on others and provoke reactions. Self-control is the way in which we moderate the impact we have on others. Empathy involves being able to put ourselves in the shoes of another person to try to understand their point of view and listening can help us to empathise more effectively. Conflict is inevitable, but there are many ways in which the results of conflict might be influenced. Co-operation offers a way of working together to achieve better conditions.

Although Goleman's ideas were discussed in the context of how children can learn to manage their own emotions and thus participate more democratically in schools, there are many lessons in his work for all of us working in settings that typically have highly emotional interpersonal relationships.

DEVELOPING PERSONAL IDENTITY AS A LEADER

Many of the issues we have discussed in this chapter contribute to the way in which you are able to develop a sense of personal identity as a leader. Many elements contribute to identity and these include:

- your approach to teamworking;
- the extent to which you respect and value others;
- your personal range of competence, including clinical, professional and managerial competence, communications, information handling and interpersonal relationships;
- your ability to learn and to develop yourself and others;
- your ability to create vision and a sense of purpose with others;
- your ability to generate passion, energy and support for action;
- the ways in which you react to pressure on yourself and others;
- the way in which you demonstrate care for the well-being and safety of others.

Our sources of energy are often closely connected with our self-esteem and confidence, and without personal energy we cannot offer leadership.

This chapter has emphasised that taking a leading role is a personal commitment. Not only do we need to consider how we develop ourselves, but we also need to contribute to the development of others. A change of role or addition of a role involves a transition that is not always easily negotiated. There is also a possibility that a new role will be more stressful than previous roles. We need to both take care of ourselves and ensure that we develop ourselves throughout our careers if we are to be effective as teamworkers and leaders.

CHAPTER 6

DEVELOPING CHANGE AGENTS

The term 'change agent' has become widely used to describe people who are able to be agents of change within their workplaces. Anybody can be a change agent and it usually involves taking a leading role. In settings where leadership is shared a normal aspect of team-working is to be asked to take a lead on some aspect of the work. Almost everyone needs to be able to be a change agent.

In this chapter we consider how individuals and teams might be developed to be comfortable in living and working through change and to be agents of change. Leadership includes responsibility for supporting others to learn and develop through the change process. We discuss attitudes and approaches to facilitating the learning and development of others.

INDIVIDUALS, GROUPS AND TEAMS

Most people working in health and care services work for at least some of the time in groups or teams, making their individual contribution to a collective activity. The main distinction between a group and a team is the way in which a team develops an identity, usually through commitment to a common purpose. Groups may become teams but teams are always groups simply because they are made up of a number of individuals. There are times for most of us when we act alone, times when we experience the greater diversity of work in groups and times when we work in teams, towards a shared goal.

Most organisations have formal and informal groups. Some of the important aspects of groups are:

- Size – It is difficult to involve everyone if a group is larger than about 10 people, but the more people, the greater the diversity, although it becomes more difficult to participate in larger groups.
- Work – Some groups exist for a long time working on fairly routine tasks and some are formed to work on a particular issue.

Groups are often expected to work on several different types of tasks and to do this may have to work in different styles. For example, some divide their meeting times into routine matters and longer discussion items.

■ Status – A group that is recognised by the organisation will be able to report and influence the organisation. Informal groups have to develop ways of bringing their issues to the attention of the organisation. Similarly, formal groups can usually call on resources and support, but informal groups have to negotiate these.

Groups can develop awareness of their processes and review the ways in which they work. If the group is to progress its work it needs to attend to both maintenance of the group and progression of its tasks.

Example 6.1: Group processes

Some of the behaviours that are needed in a group are:

Task progression	Maintenance
Proposing ideas to progress the task	Involving contributions to discussion
Building on ideas	Creating a friendly and welcoming atmosphere
Challenging ideas	Compromising and accommodating
Providing data, information, opinions	Emphasising positive feedback for individuals
Summarising, noting action points	Recognising personal feelings

These are different types of behaviour and different members of the group may need to take responsibility for the different aspects of group work, according to their individual strengths and areas of competence.

Groups are made up of individuals and sometimes the group has to consider how to respond to behaviour that does not contribute to the work of the group. Sometimes individuals have to be challenged about self-interest and groups may have to take collective responsibility about how best to use their time and energy.

There are some common problems faced by groups. Relationships in groups are sometimes stressful and people may find it difficult to contribute, particularly when groups are large. Not only are the full range of contributions lost if some group members do not contribute, but problems can emerge because only a limited range of perspectives have been identified. For example, members of a group may be unwilling to challenge someone in a more senior position or who they believe knows more than they do, but that individual's view may bring a contribution from a particular area of work that is essential to making progress. If one person in a group holds significant power over others, this is also likely to influence the freedom that group members feel to express their ideas.

People who come from similar areas of work and backgrounds are particularly prone to 'groupthink', where ideas that are familiar and welcome are accepted without examination or challenge but un-familiar or challenging ideas are rejected without open consideration. One of the main ways to avoid this is to include people in the group who are likely to bring diversity in their views. If you do this, you also need to ensure that these people are listened to and fully included in developing the group processes.

Teams have some similarities with groups but also have important differences. Group work or individual work can be less demanding than teamwork because of the interdependence of teamworking. Teams usually have to develop closer collaborative ways of working whereas groups can often be successful with a limited degree of co-operation.

Groups are useful ways of working when:

■ tasks are simple;
■ co-operation is needed more than agreement;
■ there is little need for discretion;
■ fast decisions are needed;
■ group members may have conflicting views;
■ innovative responses are needed.

Teams are more likely to be needed when:

■ tasks or problems are complex;
■ consensus decisions are essential;
■ there is a high level of choice and uncertainty;
■ high commitment of members is needed;
■ a mix of different competencies are needed;
■ members' objectives can be aligned with the task.

Teams may need to pay more attention to the balance of individual and team interactions and the ways they approach the task, mainly because of the need to agree how they will address the task. The commitment of individuals to the purpose is one of the key differ-ences between the team and the group. In a group people may co-operate without supporting the initiative with any particular enthusiasm, but in a team the shared purpose provides much of the necessary energy to enable achievement of complex outcomes.

SUPPORTING LEARNING AND DEVELOPMENT

Two important aspects of learning are different for an individual who takes a leading role. One is that you become a model of a learner for those who recognise your example as a leader, and the other is that you take on a responsibility for supporting learning, particularly the learning and development needs of those who are participating in change initiatives that you are progressing. Your attitude to learning and development, the time and energy that you invest in your own learning and development and the way in which you support others will all be influential once you are in a leading role. If you engage in critical reflective practice and share some of your reflections with your colleagues and teams, this will be influential in generating reflective approaches as a normal aspect of work. Similarly, you may be willing to share your experience of transformative learning and encourage others to recognise the extent to which such transformation can affect the whole of a person's life and not only their working lives.

Example 6.2: My reflective diaries

I start a new reflective diary whenever I start a new project that I think will be quite difficult or one that I expect to think about differently as I work through it. I go out to buy a book that I like the look of and it is rather symbolic for me as it confirms that I'm setting off into something new that I'm not sure about. The book itself becomes a companion. I tend to use it to discuss things with myself. Sometimes I just write what has happened, particularly if I'm angry or confused. I often find that just writing things down stops them buzzing in my head, so is quite a release. I go back through my notes and often find that I understand them differently after a time, so then I write about that as well. Sometimes this helps me to understand my reactions to events. It is very helpful when it stops me in my tracks and I realise that I'm repeating behaviour that wasn't successful before. I've often found that it helps me to stop and think rather than just reacting emotionally. I sometimes use the diary to work out what options I have and how to make choices. So I'd recommend trying it – but I never, ever, show my diaries to anyone else!

Carl Rogers has been influential in shaping approaches to supporting learning. He used the term 'person-centred' in working with adults to emphasise an approach that put the learner at the centre of interactions. Much of his work was in therapeutic settings and he proposed that the performance of an individual in the role of a learning facilitator depends on their possessing significant attitudinal qualities:

- realness or genuineness;
- non-possessive caring;
- prizing;
- trust;
- respect;

- empathetic understanding;
- sensitive and accurate listening.

(Rogers, 1969, pp. 106–126)

Rogers also suggested some ways in which these qualities might be demonstrated in a person-centred learning setting – see Example 6.3.

Example 6.3:   Supporting person-centred learning

Carl Rogers gave some examples of how a leader or facilitator might behave if they were facilitating learning in a way that is person-centred.

The precondition is that a leader or person who is perceived as an authority figure in the situation is sufficiently secure within herself and in her relationships with others that she experiences an essential trust in the capacity of others to think for themselves and to learn for themselves. He or she regards human beings as trustworthy. If this precondition is met, then the following aspects become possible and tend to be implemented.

- The facilitator shares responsibility for the learning process with others in the learning setting.
- The facilitator provides learning resources from within herself and her own experience, from books or materials and from community experiences.
- The learner develops his or her own programme of learning, alone or in co-operation with others.
- A facilitative learning environment is provided. This climate may spring initially from the leader but as the learning process continues, it is more and more provided by the learners for each other. Learning from each other becomes as important as learning from books or other media.
- The focus is primarily on fostering the continuing process of learning. The content of the learning, while significant, falls into a secondary place.
- The learners recognise that the discipline necessary to reach their learning goals is self-discipline and not external discipline. Self-discipline is the responsibility of the learner.
- Evaluation of the extent and significance of an individual's learning is made primarily by the learner, although this may be influenced and enriched by caring feedback from other members of the group and the facilitator.

In this growth-promoting climate, the learning tends to be deeper, proceeds at a more rapid rate and is pervasive in the life and behaviour of the learner. This is because the direction is self-chosen, the learning is self-initiated and the whole person (with feelings and passions as well as intellect) is invested in the process.

(adapted from Rogers, 1969, pp. 188–189)

You might notice that Rogers places emphasis on the importance of respecting individuals and recognising that people have individual preferences and approaches to learning. In theories about learning, these are called learning styles.

LEARNING STYLES

Honey and Mumford (1986) used the experiential learning cycle (discussed in Chapter 1, Figure 1.1) to develop a process for identifying learning styles. They identified four predominant learning styles: *activist*, *reflector*, *theorist* and *pragmatist*. These four learning styles can be illustrated by looking at a typical comment that somebody who prefers each style might make:

'I'll try anything once.' (Activist)
'I need some time to think about this.' (Reflector)
'How does that fit with the outcomes we achieved last time?' (Theorist)
'What does that mean in practice?' (Pragmatist)

Honey and Mumford believed that some people learn better in one style than another, and that some may reject certain styles. This means that we might try to use only one style for learning. If, for example, we prefer to use an activist style, we may never try to find out anything about a new situation before rushing into action. If we prefer to be reflectors, we may never get round to taking action. A theorist may prefer to carry out a lot of analysis before making a decision or taking action. A pragmatist may only be interested in ideas that have an immediate application.

We may have a preferred learning style, but this does not mean that we are able to use only one style. As you read more about each style, consider whether you do make use of a wide range of styles or whether you always choose similar approaches to learning.

Example 6.4:   Learning styles

Honey and Mumford (1986) proposed that there are four predominant learning styles.

Activists
These are open-minded, and involve themselves fully in new experiences. They are not noted for their caution, nor for their tolerance of boredom. They love short-term crisis fire-fighting, the challenge of new problems, brainstorming and finding solutions. They are weaker on implementation, consolidation and anything requiring sustained effort. They are highly sociable and like to be the centre of attention.

Reflectors
They are thoughtful and cautious, preferring to consider all possible angles, and collect as much information as possible before coming to a decision. They prefer to observe others rather than take an active role themselves, and will adopt a low profile in discussions, adding their own points only when the drift of the discussion is clear.

Theorists

They approach problems logically, step by step, and adapt and integrate their observations into complex but coherent theories. They like to know the underpinning theories before putting them into practice. They like to analyse and synthesise, and to establish basic assumptions, principles, theories and models. They are often detached, and dedicated to rational objectivity. They are uncomfortable with anything that doesn't fit into their theoretical framework, and hate subjectivity, uncertainty, lateral thinking and a flippant approach.

Pragmatists

These thrive on new ideas, provided they can put them into practice. They like to get on with things, and are confident about trying to apply new ideas. Open-ended discussions are seen as highly frustrating 'beating about the bush'. Problems and opportunities are seen as a challenge, and they are sure that there is always a better way to do anything.

These are very broad generalisations and no-one is likely to completely fit within one of these categories. You and your colleagues will have preferences about how you approach learning and you may be familiar with discussions in which everyone seems to come from different perspectives. You may have found it very frustrating if you were ready to take action but others wanted to find out more before doing anything.

As we all have preferences in how we learn, the learning style that you choose when you are teamworking or in a leading role might have implications for your colleagues. Consider how your personal preferences might seem to others whom you work with in Activity 6.1.

ACTIVITY 6.1

Allow 5 minutes.

What are the implications of your preferred learning style for you as a member or leader of a team? What impact might it have on your colleagues?

_____

_____

_____

Comments

It is not always easy to listen to views from other perspectives if we approach issues differently. It is also easy to dismiss views from people who appear to be taking issues too seriously or not seriously enough. A world that consisted only of people with one learning style would have all sorts of difficulties, but we sometimes try to restrict our discussions to those who think in similar ways to ourselves because it is more comfortable to feel that we are in agreement.

Both as a team member and a leader it is particularly important that you be able to detect important differences of opinion and to ensure that problems have been considered from different viewpoints. Therefore, some understanding of differences in learning styles can be helpful in understanding the different approaches taken by colleagues as well as in understanding yourself better.

Your approach might have a significant impact on your colleagues. If you are anxious to take action before others feel that the issues have been properly explored, you are unlikely to gain support to progress. If you seem to be delaying action because you want to find out more first, others in the team may lose confidence in your commitment to action. If people feel that you have already made up your mind, they might find it difficult to insist that you listen to them properly before rushing off to do the things that you think need to be done. You may, of course, be wrong!

The ideas behind the experiential learning cycle and learning styles can be applied to your work at any time. When you approach a new task or project, do you consider which learning style might be most helpful in gaining an initial overview? When you have completed a major piece of work, do you take the time to reflect on the experience? Do you draw out what went well or less well and reflect on reasons why things went as they did? It is from this type of reflection that we can develop our own learning from our experiences and we can use this to improve our performance next time we have to carry out a similar activity.

An understanding of experiential learning and learning styles is particularly important when you are involved in supporting others in learning and development. As the leader of a group or team you might take on responsibility for a range of development needs for the whole team and for individual members.

FORMING A TEAM TO ACHIEVE CHANGE

A team is usually formed to achieve a particular purpose. Individuals are appointed to a team because of their skills, knowledge, experience and personal qualities. The nature of the task determines to a large extent what skills, knowledge and experience are required, but consideration of personal qualities can make the difference between an effective team and one that flounders. Most of us find it more comfortable to work with people who think and behave similarly to ourselves. This can lead to a very narrow way of viewing things and Belbin's work on roles in teams (1981) identified a wide range of behaviours that can usefully contribute to the work of a team. In a team where the task involves progressing a significant change, it might be very important to ensure that there are participants who can take one or more of each of these roles.

Example 6.5:   Roles in teams progressing change

Belbin's work (1981) identified a number of significant roles in teams. These roles have positive contributions but each also has what Belbin called 'allowable weaknesses'. Each role could be linked with taking a lead on an area of the team's work:

- *innovator* – original ideas, imagination, creativity (but may be weak in communication skills and reluctant to abandon or build on ideas);
- *implementer* – turns ideas and decisions into tasks and actions (but may be inflexible and reluctant to change plans);
- *completer* – sees tasks through to completion, good on detail (but can be inclined to worry and dislike casual attitudes in others);
- *evaluator* – offers critical analysis, takes a strategic view, considers options and makes judgements (but can lack drive, warmth and imagination and can dampen morale);
- *investigator* – explores opportunities and resources from many sources, enthusiastic communicator (but can jump from one task to another and lose interest);
- *shaper* – drives the team to address the task, dynamic and challenging (but can be impatient and intolerant);
- *team maintainer* – focuses on harmony, developing ideas, listening, reducing conflict (but can be indecisive and avoid confrontation);
- *co-ordinator* – clarifies goals, promotes decision making, communicates effectively (but can be seen as manipulative and not fully contributing to the work of the team);
- *expert* – provides specialist skills or knowledge (but can be narrowly focused on their own area of work and fail to see the big picture).

Many people are strong in one or two of the roles and could also contribute in others. It can be helpful for a team to discuss who will take on each of the roles and whether they have sufficient resources or need to add members. The discussion might also consider how the team will accommodate the potential difficulties that can arise from the associated characteristics of each role. Belbin's research (1981) suggested that consistently successful teams contained a mix of these roles.

Teams that are engaged in change might need rather broader interpretations of some of these roles or other roles added in order to address some of the wider issues. Any change has the potential to affect people outside the team and often outside the area of work or organisation. The team will need someone taking a lead on consultation and negotiation with all potential stakeholders. This might fit within the co-ordinator role or might be a more broadly ambassadorial role. The information role is now more complex than when Belbin identified these roles because of the increased availability of information technology. There will be considerable information in the internal systems of many organisations and also information about benchmarking and best practice that can be important to consider before making significant changes. The person in the role of resource investigator now needs IT skills and an ability to make appropriate and competent judgements about what information will be helpful for the team as this will have to be carefully selected.

It is also questionable whether the 'allowable weaknesses' are still ones that could be accommodated within an effective team. We now expect everyone to have a good grasp of the context and the reasons for change and to contribute fully to the work that is led by others. It is usually not acceptable for someone to focus on their own agreed contribution and to ignore the parallel work, unless the team commissions a contribution as a limited expert input. We expect team members to take a more holistic view of their involvement in a team than these roles may suggest. We expect responsibility to be shared.

DEVELOPING A TEAM TO ACHIEVE CHANGE

There are two aspects to team development; development of the team as a whole and development of the individuals who are members of the team. Team development includes the processes that are used by the team and the team performance in progressing the tasks.

A helpful model of team development is one developed by Tuckman and Jensen (1977) which sets out stages through which a team usually moves in becoming able to perform effectively. The five stages – forming, storming, norming, performing, adjourning – describe the internal dynamics of a team as it develops ways of working together. In a team where leadership is shared and the focus is on change we can consider the implications of each of these stages (see Example 6.6). One of the implications of this model is that performance is delayed until several stages have been successfully negotiated. In many settings today we would expect early results and would be reluctant to accept that a team could not perform effectively more quickly than this model suggests. Although the model has always allowed that teams may progress forwards and backwards through the stages, we would now expect a more parallel process of tasks being achieved while the team dynamics are collectively managed by the team membership.

Example 6.6:   Leading in a team of change agents

Five stages of team development were identified by Tuckman and Jensen (1977). This model can be useful in thinking about the stages in a team in which everyone shares responsibility for progressing the purpose and in which change is a particular concern.

Forming

This stage in the original model is one in which the team deals with hopes and fears, clarification of purpose and roles, and development of interpersonal relationships. One of the earliest tasks is also to consider whether the membership is appropriate and sufficient for the purpose and whether anyone else should be added. Alongside this, some agreement about process needs to be made so that the team anticipates and prepares ways of enabling a variety of views to be shared and how to manage disagreements. Although there will always be a need to find out more, team members should all be able to begin work from this stage.

Storming

This stage is where conflict surfaces and disruption can prevent progress. It often helps a team to consider its basic values and principles. If the team agrees to value and respect diverse views, disagreement becomes a way of reviewing perspectives. In any change situation the views of all those involved are important in determining whether progress will be supported or blocked. This model of team development is so well known now that team members might use it to help them to work through their own processes in a way that ensures that they take care to acknowledge the range of perspectives that relate to their intended change. Although the team might find that it can avoid too much disruption in working through this stage of team development, reviewing different views is not a one-off activity. Every aspect of the team's work may raise issues that have not yet been considered. A robust process needs to be developed and maintained by the team to ensure that wide consultation accompanies its progress in parallel with achievement of the team's tasks.

Norming

At this stage the team settles into agreed routine ways of working. In progressing change, however, the processes that have been agreed for the early stages of an initiative may not be the best, as time moves on and situations change. It can be a constraint for a team to develop norms that inhibit change within the team and its ways of working. The balance of the team dynamics and progress towards achievement of the purpose may need to be revisited frequently to ensure that the team is not putting too much attention into maintaining itself at the cost of progressing the task.

Performing

This is the stage at which the team is working efficiently towards its goals. As in the previous stages, nothing stands still and the situation constantly changes. The only way to be sure of effective performance is to monitor and review regularly against targets. The processes that are needed here are detailed management routines and these are not always the approaches that people oriented towards achieving change welcome. Everyone needs to be engaged in the routine monitoring activities if the reviews of progress are to be meaningful.

Adjourning

One of the characteristics of a team is that it has a limited life that completes with the achievement of its purpose. If members of the team have enjoyed working together and found the work satisfying, there is often some reluctance to break up the team. However, with people who are interested in change, there will also be an attraction in moving on to the next challenge. It is helpful if some attention is paid to closure by ensuring that team members have all given each other feedback where appropriate. Achievements can be recorded in appraisals and other documentation. It is important that learning as a team and as individuals is discussed and noted, so that people are able to use the experience gained from this team when they move into new roles.

There may be areas of team development to address that are more concerned with the nature of the task than the processes. For example, the team might benefit from briefings about particular aspects of the proposed initiative. A team that is working to improve the access to a hospital in terms of public and private transport in a geographic area might want to have briefings about current services and the degree of flexibility for change. For example, they might have presentations from each of the public service areas (probably buses and trains) and from other transport providers including taxi services, voluntary organisations and social services. They might hold a consultation meeting about the use of private cars and parking issues. They might also want to consult about the environmental impact of their ideas for change. The local government authority would have an interest in the initiative, as would other health providers and social services. It can be surprising how many stakeholders there are in an initiative that may be prompted by a local problem.

Specific development needs for change agents will include knowledge of change processes and experience in application of techniques in diagnosing situations, developing support for proposals and direction and implementing change.

Team development needs might also include some of the formal management processes of monitoring and recording progress and managing informal and formal communications (including use of technology). Individuals in the team will probably also have a wide range of personal development needs.

DEVELOPING INDIVIDUALS AS CHANGE AGENTS

Individual development includes identification of learning and development needs, personal development planning and supporting development plans. Most teams will have some members who have some knowledge and experience about these things and others who have little experience of developing themselves and others. There is an opportunity to offer development in supporting the learning and development of others through pairing in the team. If all members are to use the team's work as a developmental opportunity, it can be helpful to gain skills in supporting others as this will be an essential part of their future as change agents. Similarly, there will be opportunities to widen experience by taking on unfamiliar roles, including perhaps chairing meetings, taking on liaison roles, gathering and presenting information to the team and working with people from unfamiliar areas.

Example 6.7:   Key behaviours in successful change leaders

Sue Richards has identified some key competencies associated with successful change leaders of modernisation in public services:

1 Focus staff on the strategic purposes to be achieved so that they are aware of why they are being asked to work in a particular way.
2 Listen hard to staff to get to the real issues that must be sorted out.
3 Be able to work outside the traditional boundaries of the organisation, able to listen to members of the community and engage the public as partners in delivering better outcomes.
4 Give the highest priority to professional development because change in professional settings must have legitimacy with the professional culture.
5 Work well with leaders of local services, and build partnerships to establish seamless service across boundaries.
6 Give priority to achieving results. Stick to the purpose.
7 Use the power of information to unblock the road to change. This fits with a culture that is open rather than hidden.
8 Use project-based working to enable individuals and teams to contribute to performance improvement.
9 Talk and tell the story of change creatively and incessantly, help staff to make sense of the complex multi-layered reality of what is happening.
(adapted from Wooldridge and Wallace, 2002, pp. 28–29)

One of the tools that is particularly helpful for individuals is a Personal Development Plan (PDP). There are many formats for these, but the elements are much the same. They usually set out what you need to learn, how you will do it and how you will be able to prove that you have learnt it. For example, you might have as an objective that you want to learn to take a leading role. This involves quite a complex range of competence and skills, so you might want to spell out the ones that are most important for you to work on. This is also not an easy area to plan for learning because of its complexity. You would probably have to use a number of different approaches. These might include shadowing someone in a leading role and discussing it with them, acting up in a leading role with the support of a mentor and perhaps a coach and reflecting on the experience and perhaps studying through structured reading or a formal course. You might address specific skills in ways that involved learning how to perform the skill under guidance and then applying the skill in a suitable situation. In all cases, you would also have to think about how you will know when you have learnt it – what will you be able to do that you cannot do at the moment?

The skills and processes of supporting development at work are well covered in the literature of human resource management. These and general management skills and techniques can be found in Martin and Henderson (2001).

EMPOWERING CHANGE AGENTS

Once individuals are confident teamworkers who have some experience of progressing a significant change, they will still need some support to be able to work effectively in continuing implementation of changes or in new initiatives. A key issue for anyone seeking to initiate change is to ensure that you are able to negotiate agreement to progress your ideas. This requires skills in presenting ideas, securing support, negotiation and political awareness. There are also practicalities in checking (and perhaps in challenging) your level of authority for key areas such as finance, staffing and quality. You need to be able to consult and to listen carefully to different views and to check out your interpretation after consultations. You will also need to be clear about your accountability and who will support you and confirm that you are progressing in the agreed direction.

Change often provokes strong emotions, however inevitable it may seem that some action must be taken. Individuals who take action and are seen to be progressing change can attract more attention than they are used to coping with and can also sometimes find hostility directed to them in a personal way. Change agents need the support of peers but also of those in organisations who have the formal authority to provide resources and back-up. Without such empowering support, individuals find it very difficult to make even local and limited changes.

We should not doubt that investment in individuals and teamworking produces desirable outcomes in health and social care services. In a study of sixty-one hospitals in England, recent research demonstrated that the Human Resource Management approaches had a direct relationship with the mortality of patients. Specifically, the research found that:

- appraisal has the strongest relationship with patient mortality;
- the extent of teamworking in hospitals is also strongly related to patient mortality;
- sophistication of training policies is linked to lower patient mortality.

Michael West, who lead the research, comments:

> If you have in place HR practices that focus effort and skill; if you develop people's skills; and if you encourage co-operation, collaboration, innovation and synergy in teams; and you do this for most if not all employees in the organisation, the whole system functions more effectively and performs better as a result. The effects show across the board, even in measures of performance as fundamental as patient deaths in hospitals. If the receptionists, porters, ancillary staff, secretaries, nurses, managers, and, yes, the doctors are working effectively in a system the system as a whole will function effectively.
>
> (West, 2002, pp. 12–14)

Staff development and empowerment is a life and death issue.

This chapter has focused on how individuals can be developed to be change agents. We have reviewed some of the issues raised in working in groups and teams in terms of the activities that will progress change. Support and development of others is a key role of change agents, but we also need awareness of ourselves and the impact of our behaviour on others. Much of the discussion in this chapter may have provided ideas for personal development. The evidence that staff development directly affects the lives of service users confirms that we should invest in development.

CHAPTER 7

LEADING LEARNING

As a leader in health and social care, you need to be aware of the use of evidence in making decisions about any course of action. We look at the nature of evidence and ways of judging how much confidence to have in using it to support our decisions. We take a look at how evidence is generated through different processes of research and enquiry and how we might form a view about the value of the results presented.

We then look at how a leader might contribute to organisational learning. Health and social care services are often interdisciplinary and inter-professional and also sometimes inter-agency. People work together who have very different backgrounds and different learning experience and hence often have different views of the world. Those in leadership roles can help to develop shared understandings of the issues in different areas of work.

We complete the chapter by reviewing what is known about learning and knowledge management in organisations and the contribution that can be made by those in leading roles. We explore some of the ideas that have been successful in facilitating and managing learning in health and social care settings and ways in which leaders can promote and support learning.

'real change and the ability to adapt to change within organisations, in industry, and changes in the world at large, *has to start within each individual*. . . . Successful leaders will have to be willing to learn and constantly be aware of the way people think, how and why they behave in certain ways, how they learn and unlearn, and how to tap into their personal energy.' (April, Macdonald and Vriesendorp, 2000, p. 48)

LEARNING FROM EVIDENCE

Any leader in health and care services has to handle a lot of information and needs to develop skills to help them to manage information effectively. Do you know what is meant by an evidence-based approach? This term is now widely used in health professions and is closely related to learning through enquiry. There are implications of this approach for you as a learner because you need to have some appreciation of what evidence is and how evidence can be used to help to make decisions.

The evidence-based approach to practice has arisen from recognition of the tension between certainty and uncertainty in many areas of practice, including clinical practice:

> Perhaps the most important skill for any health care professional to master in their career is the ability to recognise and handle clinical uncertainty: uncertainty, as it is manifested in the range of unpredictable and often untimely conditions presented by our patients in wards, outpatients, and in the consulting room; but also uncertainty about one's own skill, expertise and knowledge base.
>
> The ongoing tension between certainty over uncertainty is the driving force of the evidence-based practice movement. Its central philosophy is one of never taking for granted one's own practice, and by using a structured, problem-based approach each practitioner can logically manoeuvre their way through the obstacle race of clinical decision making.
>
> (Kitson in Dawes *et al.*, 1999, Foreword)

In that second paragraph there are several ideas that support taking a critical reflective approach to practice. If we never take our own practice for granted we must always be open to changing how we do things and to developing our understanding of why we do things as we do. If we use a structured approach to identifying and solving problems, we are able to approach each situation equipped with a process that will help us to assess what we find, to plan an appropriate response, to take action and then to evaluate whether the problem has been solved. Does this sound familiar? It is a process that links closely with the experiential learning cycle discussed in Chapter 1.

The evidence-based approach is now used widely in health care because it links practice into the increasingly important databases of evidence about what is known about different options and whether there is a recommended best practice. The databases are developing and there is not as yet evidence relating to every area of practice. However, wherever there is evidence to support a recommendation of best practice, everyone will expect health professionals to be familiar with the recommendation and to follow the guidelines.

For health professionals this approach brings responsibilities rather different from the traditional ones. It is no longer sufficient to study for a few years to become a registered practitioner and to expect at that point that you will know enough to practice effectively for the rest of your career. Now it is widely acknowledged that all health professionals and other health and care workers must commit themselves to lifelong learning. You can expect to be learning throughout your career. This is why it is important to be an effective and confident learner who is able to learn independently.

THE NATURE OF EVIDENCE

Let's look more closely at what is meant by evidence-based practice. We gather evidence for our practice from many sources. If you have been in health care practice for some time already, you will have experience to draw on that will often inform your practice. You may also use other sources to gather evidence, for example textbooks and journal articles. You will also be aware of how difficult it is to find time to read all the information that might be available.

If we are to base our decisions on evidence or present evidence in support of our claims, we need to understand the nature of evidence. It would be very reassuring to be able to say that a claim is true whenever there is evidence to support it. However, evidence may or may not be convincing in its use to support a claim. We are not able to use evidence as a truth that cannot be challenged, because evidence might be used in a number of different ways for a number of different purposes. Evidence is relative. It contributes to making something clearer or more visible. Evidence is often used to support a statement of belief, to offer proof. However, people hold different beliefs and these are closely related to the different values and attitudes that we all hold. The nature of the evidence and how it has been collected are very important in considering how evidence can be used effectively.

Evidence is usually in the form of data relating to the issue under investigation. It may consist of physical things or of statements and opinions. This raises a number of issues.

1. Data is not information until we have interpreted it in some way. Data might consist of different types of things, for example statistics, numbers, written statements, oral statements or photographs. If you want to prove that you are competent in carrying out an activity you might present evidence including:

   ■ memos relating to a particular occasion or event;
   ■ formal papers that you have prepared;
   ■ witness statements from people who say that they have seen you carry out the activity successfully;
   ■ your own statement explaining how you did it;

   or other things that you believe support your claim. However, your belief that the evidence supports the claim will not necessarily be sufficient to convince others.

2. Interpretation is often personal and subjective because it relies on our knowledge and experience. For example, you might believe that you have acted in an efficient and effective way in carrying out your activities. However, your judgement is related to the experience and knowledge that you have. A more experienced person with wider knowledge would be able to make a judgement that

draws on a greater number of examples giving a wider comparison. This might corroborate your opinion or might present challenges. This is one of the reasons for the increasing interest in making comparisons between achievements of standards and considering what 'good practice' or 'best value' might comprise. Interpretation is based on judgement. Judgement is about comparing things and coming to a conclusion based on the comparison.

3. Last, data have been collected before they are presented as evidence and the way in which data are collected will have shaped the data.

ACTIVITY 7.1

Allow 5 minutes.

Imagine that it is widely known that the reception area for your service has to be moved to a new location which is yet to be agreed. Several members of your team come to you with a suggestion that the reception area for your service should be transferred to a site close to the new shopping centre. They are sure that this is a wonderful opportunity and that it would be much more convenient for everyone. They show you evidence that service users have been consulted and agree that it is a good idea. Would you be convinced? Make notes of anything that you would want to ask them.

_____

_____

_____

_____

You would want to know how they collected the evidence that they are presenting to support their argument. If they are so convinced by this idea, they may not have looked for any opposing ideas or even noticed if any objections were presented to them. There is a possibility that people will only seek out and present data that can be interpreted to support their ideas. You would also probably want to know whom they had consulted, for example, had they sought the views of different service users, including those with mobility difficulties? Had different age groups been consulted? Had representatives from partner or linked services been consulted? Had support services been consulted? Had they considered the financial aspects and the organisational strategy? Had you and other managers been consulted? You would form an opinion about the extent to which you could have confidence in the evidence presented.

Evidence is data interpreted as information and used as proof to support an argument. If we are to be convinced by the argument, we need to be convinced that this evidence is acceptable. There are some tests that can be applied to help you to decide whether evidence is acceptable:

- Is it sufficient?
- Is it authentic?
- Is it valid?
- Is it current?

SUFFICIENT EVIDENCE

Is the evidence enough to support the claim that is made? If it is claimed that 100 service users have been asked for their views you would want to see that there were 100 responses. However, this would still not in itself be enough to convince you that this was evidence that you could trust. You might want to know that all the different categories of service users were represented amongst the 100 that had responded. For example, if you think about change of location for a service reception, you might want to see more responses from service users who might find it difficult to use a different location for any reason.

AUTHENTIC EVIDENCE

Is this evidence what it is claimed to be? In the case of our example, have the staff who are presenting this evidence really collected 100 responses from a range of service users? Were all those who responded users of your service? Does it matter whether they were current or past users or whether they had never had cause to use your services but would be entitled to if the need arose? Who actually collected the data? Are you seeing the information in the same form as it was when collected or has it been analysed and interpreted in any way? If so, is it still representative of the original data or has it been interpreted to present the proposal in a better light?

VALID EVIDENCE

Does this evidence demonstrate what is claimed? Using our example, how was the evidence collected from the 100 respondents? Did they understand what was being asked? Were they asked whether they would like the suggested new location or were they asked which of a number of possible new locations they would prefer? The answers might well differ if the questions are asked in different ways. How closely does the evidence represent what service users really think? How real or truthful is the evidence? Does this evidence really prove what is claimed? Could it be interpreted in any other way? Is too much being claimed on too little evidence? Have opposing views been sought?

CURRENT EVIDENCE

Is the evidence up to date? This is important in situations where there is rapid change and when opinions might change. What people think about an issue will depend on whether there has been any recent event that might have changed attitudes.

It is not easy to produce evidence that is convincing when you are investigating an issue that concerns a number of people or groups of people with potentially different interests.

USING RESEARCH STUDIES

Much of the information that is helpful in making decisions about practice in health and care comes from research studies. There are many different types of research and it is important to understand something about the approaches used by researchers if you are to be able to form your own views about how much confidence to place in the evidence that is presented in research results.

One of the research approaches that has been very influential in developing medical and clinical knowledge is a technique known as 'randomised controlled trial'. A randomised controlled trial (RCT) is a way of evaluating the success of a particular treatment. The experimental treatment is given to one group of patients and a placebo is given to another group. All of the patients involved must agree to be part of the trial and to either be given the treatment or not. Ideally the people giving the treatment, having the treatment, and evaluating the clinical effect will also not know whether the experimental treatment or a placebo is being given. At the end of the course of treatment the outcome is assessed by comparing the two groups to see whether the experimental treatment produced better results than the placebo treatment.

There has been a considerable increase in the number of randomised controlled trials that are carried out and it would be difficult and time-consuming to search these to come to some conclusion about how to treat any particular condition. There is now a lot of help for practitioners who need to draw on this research so that each individual does not have to make an appraisal of all of the available evidence before deciding how to act. There are now libraries that present reviews of randomised trials in clear and straightforward language so that practitioners can quickly access the latest conclusions that can be drawn from all the available and reliable research. The Cochrane Library of Systematic Reviews is one of these resources.

Example 7.1: The Cochrane Library

Good evidence is needed for high-quality health care, but finding good evidence is not easy. The problem lies in accessing the evidence that is there. Unfortunately no one can keep up to date with the relevant evidence in their field because every year the volume of this evidence increases. Worse still, the major bibliographic databases available to most health care professionals (e.g. Cinhal, Medline) cover less than half the world's literature and are biased towards English-language publications. The average researcher will probably find only a fraction of the evidence using the major databases and even when found, the evidence may be unreliable, the quality of the studies being poor and the results biased. Also, much evidence is unpublished and this may be of great importance.

The Cochrane Library aims to solve these problems and is generally recognised to be the best source of reliable evidence about the effects of health care. Volunteers act as reviewers and give attention to one area of health care interventions. The reviews concentrate on controlled trials and develop highly structured and systematic reviews of the evidence. Data from studies are carefully examined and analysed using specially developed software. The results are then published in electronic form in the Cochrane Library.

You might be interested to look at an abstract of the review conducted by Arrowsmith who is a reviewer for the Cochrane Library: 'Removal of nail polish and finger rings by scrubbed personnel to prevent surgical infection'. Do you know whether these staff should remove rings and nail polish? Check what evidence was found about whether people working in operating theatres can wear nail polish or finger rings without increasing post-operative wound infection rates. The abstract is free of charge on http://www.cochrane.org/cochrane/reabstr/abidx.htm. To access the full text of the review you will need to consult the Cochrane Library on CD-ROM or via the Internet. It is available on subscription, updated four times per year and you may find your employer already subscribes to it.

(Vickie Arrowsmith, School of Health and
Social Welfare at the Open University)

You might like to look carefully at the Cochrane Library so that you become familiar with the range and type of reports that it contains and find out whether there is any evidence that relates to your area of practice.

Research methods vary according to the questions that are asked and the settings in which the research is conducted. Not all research is or should be carried out with the large numbers of participants that are necessary for randomised controlled trials because the method has to be appropriate for the purpose of the research. It is also not always appropriate to use quantitative methods because many types of knowledge do not involve things that can be meaningfully counted.

Qualitative research methods allow us to carry out enquiries that explore the experience of people in contexts. Questions about interactions, processes and activities are often best explored through qualitative methods. For example, comparisons can be made through use of case studies (Yin, 1994) and individual case studies can explore the features of a particular work area or organisation. Action research (Stringer, 1996) can be a good way to approach enquiry in a particular situation over a period of time. Stringer (1996) also discusses participative approaches that can be appropriate when group members work together to explore their collective experience. Other useful books that discuss the choices we make in research are Reason and Rowan's *Human Inquiry* (1981), Easterby-Smith, Thorpe and Lowe's *Management Research* (1991), Denzin and Lincoln's *The Landscape of Qualitative Research* (1998) and Greenfield's *Research Methods for Postgraduates* (2002).

The most important consideration in planning your own research or evaluating the research of others is whether the research method chosen was appropriate for seeking answers to the research questions. If so, you can then consider the extent to which the questions were answered and how much confidence you can have in the answers. The criteria for your judgement are the same as the criteria that you can use to judge any evidence. You might ask whether the range of the research was sufficient. If the questions involved only a small community in a boundaried setting the study may only need to be small-scale and only involve those in that setting. Questions that relate to larger-scale settings might be addressed satisfactorily if a careful selection of representative elements in the setting are used. Authenticity is important and will need to be considered. Is the information authentic and was it collected in an appropriate way from the appropriate people? Is it valid in terms of what it claims as findings? Even if these criteria are satisfied, you must ask how recent the research is and to what extent the findings might still be useful in informing current thinking.

LEARNING IN AN ORGANISATION

There has been an increasing interest in how organisations develop and how this relates to ways in which individuals learn and develop. Organisational learning has the potential to include:

- building awareness in an organisation of how learning can be shared and transferred to inform different areas of work;
- awareness of how what is learnt from projects and change initiatives can be used to inform future developments;
- management of knowledge within an organisation so that it is available to support continuous development.

It also includes understanding of learning and development processes and how learning together can contribute to working together. Once again, learning is associated with the ability to change and to transform when necessary.

In 1970 Donald Shon talked of organisations as potential 'learning systems' capable of continual transformation (cited in Pedler, Burgoyne, Boydell and Welshman, 1990, p. 14). Later Shon developed these ideas with Argyris and described 'double loop learning' in which an organisation engages in learning systematically and applies the learning to change itself by challenging its current assumptions, norms and values. They were, however, unable to find an example of an organisation that did this (Argyris and Shon, 1978, p. 312). Continuous change of this nature runs counter to many of the accepted notions of good practice in organisations. For example, long-term strategic, financial and marketing planning and traditions of bureaucratic procedures all rely on some degree of stability.

Bob Garratt developed some approaches to a learning organisation (1987) and the team of Pedler, Burgoyne and Boydell presented a collection of ideas relating to a concept of a learning company in 1991, recognising that it may be a dream and not immediately available:

> The Learning Company is a vision of what might be possible. It is not brought about simply by training individuals; it can only happen as a result of *learning at the whole organisational level*:
>
>> A Learning Company is an organisation that facilitates the learning of all its members and continuously transforms itself.
>
>> This is the dream – that we can design and create organisations which are capable of adapting, changing, developing and transforming themselves in response to the needs, wishes and aspirations of people, inside and outside. Such companies will always be realising their assets without predatory takeovers; they will be able to flex without hiring a new Top Man; they will be able to avoid the sudden and massive restructurings that happen after years of not noticing the signals.
>
> (Pedler, Burgoyne and Boydell, 1991, p. 1)

They suggest that there are three perspectives that are particularly significant in whether an organisation can become a learning entity:

■ the ideas, the visions and images of the company;
■ the life stage and stage of development of the organisation;
■ the cultural and economic context in which the company exists.

Although they think that ideas are a strong force in shaping practice within an organisation, they recognise that organisations develop traditions and expectations that may inhibit learning by subduing challenges to existing practice. Leaders in organisations have a role in helping to develop learning within their organisation and areas of work by being open to new ideas and by looking for ways of sharing innovations in practice and new knowledge.

CONTRIBUTING TO A LEARNING CULTURE

Learning is personal for individuals, as it is about how we make meaning and develop understanding from our own perspectives. Similarly, in an organisation or an area of work, learning is an aspect of the culture, the ways in which people normally behave and interact together. If learning is valued and respected, it is much easier to build time and attention into day-to-day work to allow opportunities to share and capture learning so that others can benefit from the learning of individuals and groups.

The term 'knowledge management' is widely used now, but often refers only to the ways in which an organisation manages its data and information systems. A wider interpretation is to think about the knowledge that resides in individuals and teams, the 'know-how' that enables them to work efficiently and effectively. Many people make continuous innovations and improvements in the ways they carry out their work and these can make the difference between effective and up-to-date performance and performance that is barely adequate because it is no longer fully suitable for the context or setting. As our working settings constantly change, we need to make appropriate and often subtle changes in how we work in them. Not everyone notices the need to do this or believes that they should be revising practices and procedures that were adequate five or ten years ago.

'One thing that all managers know is that many of the best ideas never get put into practice ... because they conflict with deeply held internal images of how the world works, images that limit us to familiar ways of thinking and acting. That is why the discipline of managing mental models – surfacing, testing, and improving our internal pictures of how the world works – promises to be a major breakthrough for building learning organizations.' (Senge, 1990, p. 174)

Effective knowledge management in an organisation enables it to identify which individuals and teams are performing in a way that provides an example of good practice and then encourages ways of sharing what it is that contributes to creating a better performance. This is not easy, as any challenge to performance can raise anxiety and defensive responses. A culture that encourages learning might approach ideas about best practice in a spirit of enquiry, asking why it is that in some times and places we consistently do better than in others. Although there may be significant differences in resources and morale, there are usually also differences in processes. Some of the most useful sharing of knowledge is in this 'know-how' area where innovations have produced better ways of doing things.

There are different ways of sharing knowledge and the choice depends on the type of knowledge to be shared and the knowledge and experience of those wanting to learn. The method of sharing has to be appropriate for the individuals and teams offering to share and learning from others. We will consider the methods that might be used to share and the conditions that help or hinder in use of each method.

Databases

There are increasing numbers of databases that report initiatives that represent good practice and innovation in areas of health and social care practice. Larger organisations can create internal databases to enable their own staff to hear about local developments. It is, perhaps, the first stage in enabling sharing of knowledge to simply make new knowledge available. It is not always easy, though, for people to see how they might be influenced by new ideas. It is widely recognised that transfer of knowledge is one of the key difficulties to overcome if an organisation is to be effective in managing knowledge.

Databases are helpful in raising awareness of improvements in practice if people access them and consider the implications for their own areas of work. The use of databases is limited, however, by the extent to which people are able to recognise the innovative elements of the initiative reported and also by the existing knowledge of the reader. If people using a database already have knowledge and experience in the same or a related field, they are much more likely to be able to make use of the ideas than those who are encountering the field for the first time.

There are also limitations to the type of knowledge that can be presented effectively in a database. It is an appropriate medium if the issues are easy to explain clearly in writing. Even so, there is no guarantee that those reading the explanation will understand the ideas in a similar way to those who wrote the item. There is no opportunity with a database to ask questions or to check out your understanding, so there are limits that often need to be overcome by using other approaches.

Interactive exchange at a distance

Use of telephones, e-mail, videos and video conferencing enables ideas to be exchanged effectively without face-to-face meetings. A fairly simple innovation that is difficult to explain in words might be effectively shared through demonstration that could be recorded as a video or CD–ROM. This is a good way to explain procedures that involve physical activities, especially when the innovation is a different way of carrying out the procedure. A demonstration with a verbal explanation can be very effective in sharing a practical innovation when learners already have enough knowledge and experience to follow the description. If there is likely to be a need to ask questions or to check out understanding, then it might be necessary to make links by phone or e-mail to enable some discussion.

This approach is increasingly being used in health organisations to enable consultation with experts at a distance. For example, X-ray images or even a patient might be viewed in a video conference so that consultation can be held without the need for a face-to-face meeting that might be very difficult to arrange with geographic and time considerations. An expert might even be invited to support an intervention in practice by joining the event through video conferencing.

More simply, telephone contact allows conversations to be held about issues that might include sharing of information, advice and reassurance. For example, the NHS Direct service has become very popular as a way of providing instant access to information and advice for service users who no longer need to always go to local services in person.

The advantages of interactive contact include the possibility of asking questions and checking understanding. If a visual contact is made, there is also the potential to see how someone carries out a procedure. More complicated initiatives can be discussed through use of a range of technologies for communication at a distance.

Working alongside

Many innovations in health and care services are in complex settings where activities have to be adapted to some extent to accommodate the specific needs of people and settings. Although descriptions and discussions of initiatives that improve practice in such settings can interest and motivate people in other places who would like to improve their own practice, it is often very difficult to understand the issues at a distance. Rather than struggle to try to explain the complexity, it can be much more effective to arrange to visit the team that have developed a different way of working so that they can see it in action in its own setting. Such visits also enable some discussion of the differences in context and the ways in which the ideas might be adapted to work in different settings.

Another approach is to ask those who have developed a new expertise to visit you to explain and demonstrate to your team. This can be very helpful when the situations are similar enough for ideas to be transferred fairly easily once they are understood.

Enabling some of the learning team to work alongside the team who developed the innovation might better provide an effective learning experience for complicated innovations. This would provide the learners with direct experience over a short period of time. The learners could then rejoin their home teams with the knowledge and experience of having used the new processes and also with contacts from their placement who could continue to be available for consultation if needed.

Example 7.2:   Sharing 'know-how'

A team of nurses in a specialist service working with people who had diabetes had secured resources to run a clinic through which they would be able to work more closely with their patients and help them to take a more active role in managing their own conditions.

One of the nurses had excited the others in the team when she had come across an article in a database that described an initiative that seemed to have developed an effective way of providing diverse and flexible services in this sort of clinic. The nurses had been discussing how they might offer more personal support and advice and felt that patients would both welcome and benefit from an extension of the services. The group had been supported by others in the organisation to develop a proposal and to secure resources that established the facilities and a pilot service. They then realised that they had not considered very carefully exactly how they would work differently. They became rather worried about how to design the service to be sure that it would be effective in offering greater benefits than they had been able to offer in their traditional approach.

At this point they realised that they needed to discuss their ideas with the people who had developed the innovative approach that had stimulated their ideas. They managed to make phone contact from the information given in the database article. The team who had developed the innovation were delighted to find that others were interested and immediately invited them to visit and see how their services worked. This led to an exchange through which several members of each team swapped roles for a week to work alongside the other teams.

These teams stayed in close contact because they realised that they were developing some new ways of working that might have potential benefits in other settings. Once they were confident that they had ironed out the initial difficulties, they were able to share their ideas more widely to support similar initiatives in different settings.

Sharing knowledge and 'know-how' in these ways can be very motivating and satisfying for the staff involved. To some extent, people can develop learning experiences of this nature even if the culture of their organisation is less than encouraging, but approaching others for learning support can often feel like asking a favour. If an organisation is serious about facilitating and encouraging the sharing of knowledge, there are some steps that can be taken to establish a helpful climate.

Nancy Dixon suggested four key principles for enabling knowledge transfer:

- Design the system as an exchange between peers. Avoid implying that 'the best' is to be transferred to the 'less capable'.
- Knowledge resides in people. People often need to be in the situation in order to recall and apply the knowledge and to share it with others.
- The source of the knowledge should be involved in translating it into the new situation whenever possible. They have the knowledge and experience to draw together seemingly unconnected ideas to form solutions in new settings.

■ Name the knowledge transfer system to legitimise it and enable people to use it without seeming to be asking for help or favours.

(adapted from Dixon, 2000, p. 39)

If knowledge management is to be taken seriously within an organisation, it needs to be widely understood, adequately resourced and built into day-to-day practice. Those who provide information services need to work with those who work in human resource development and training, so that blended approaches can be developed.

Those who want to work in settings in which learning is respected and facilitated can be leaders in creating these conditions. The arguments become compelling when examples of improvements are used to demonstrate what sharing learning has achieved. Support for learning has to compete with other imperatives for a fair share of available resources, so it is usually necessary not only to convince people of the need to develop a learning culture but also to provide examples of the benefits such a culture can bring.

CHAPTER 8

BEING AWARE

This chapter is about how leaders can become more aware of the need for change in themselves and in their settings. Awareness is more than noticing – it involves recognition of patterns and development of understanding about our surroundings and ourselves. We need to be aware if we are to contribute to the development and shaping of better health and care services.

Change is stimulated in many different ways and is now often considered to be a constant state in organisations. Health and social care organisations are complex because of the range of needs that these services attempt to address, the number of people that the services attempt to help and the interdependence of the many organisations and agencies that collaborate to deliver services. There are demands made on health and care that stimulate change in services. There is also demand for change from within service areas. People who are aware of the pressures to change, but who are also aware of the interdependent nature of complex service provision, have the potential to be successful change agents in health and care settings.

In this chapter some of the pressures for change in health and care services are reviewed and the potential for leaders to take a proactive role is considered. Changes can be widespread and significant throughout an organisation but can also be quite small and mostly focused on one area of work, although there are normally some implications for other areas of work. Some models of change are discussed, together with some ideas about how to focus on an area of work in which change might be led proactively. The chapter concludes by bringing the process of leading change into the context of change in complex services and by taking a systems overview of change. This model provides an overview of the content of the following chapters.

AWARENESS

'Taking a hard look into the mirror [of the present moment] is like listening inwardly and finding out what you need to let go of and what you need to develop. Bring aware is a fundamental mode of existence in the world, a prerequisite for aliveness, for authentic self-expression and authentic relationships.' (April, Macdonald and Vriesendorp, 2000, p. 124)

Awareness is about noticing what is happening in the world around you. It includes observing and listening, being sensitive to the inter-actions in your immediate surroundings. It also includes noticing what is changing in the wider world and understanding how that might have an impact on you, your colleagues and those who use your services. It also means understanding and accepting the impli-cations of the ways in which your own actions affect the responses and actions of others.

Awareness of self means knowing yourself well enough to under-stand what you can contribute in different situations and what strengths you have. It also involves understanding the impressions that you make on others by the ways in which you communicate and behave. Many people learn self-awareness by seeking feedback from others and reflecting on this. Many people find that participating in action learning sets can raise self-awareness through informal and supportive peer group discussion. Formal appraisal processes can also be enlightening and lead to support for self-development.

Awareness of the issues that often arise during a significant trans-formation can both prepare you to plan carefully and help you to notice signs of potential disruption before things get out of hand. Transformation is significant change. To achieve a transformation we have to change the ways we think and behave, although the focus will often be on achieving better results. Awareness of change includes understanding some of the ways that change can be achieved within organisations and the importance of the impact that change can have on individuals and groups. Significant change requires people to learn to think and act differently. This is rarely easy and sometimes very challenging for people.

WHAT DRIVES CHANGE?

Whether we like change or not, we are all caught up in a never-ending cycle of change in our organisations and in our lives. Some people welcome change and enjoy the uncertainty it often brings, thinking that it offers new challenges and opportunities. Others are cautious about change, fearing that something valued will be altered or lost or that risk brings unnecessary stress. Some are sceptical about the promised benefits of change. Sometimes our feelings about change relate to the position we find ourselves in. It is useful to reflect on how you react to change and whether your reactions are related to how changes are introduced.

ACTIVITY 8.1

Allow 10 minutes

Think about a change that you have experienced at work.

How did you feel about the change?

Were you involved in initiating the change or was it forced on you?

Were you able to influence the change at all?

Was it clear why the change needed to take place?

Did you understand exactly what would happen?

Was there any misunderstanding or disagreement?

Did it achieve the results that were intended?

Did it change your work in any way?

Was it stressful or threatening for you?

Was anything lost that you valued?

Was anything gained?

These are examples of the questions that individuals often ask about change in organisations. As you thought about these questions you may have had quite vivid recollections of how you felt, particularly if you experienced something that felt like an injustice or that led to the loss of something that you valued. Even if you recognised that the change had to happen, you may have taken some time to see the value of what was gained. You may have experienced different reactions to change, depending on whether you were involved in carrying out the change and able to shape it in ways to accommodate your concerns or whether the change was imposed on you without consultation. Change often touches quite deeply on our emotions, sometimes over issues that we did not realise we cared about.

It is often said that change is a constant in our working lives. As change has the potential to cause emotional reactions, our working lives can feel very stressful and uncertain. In health and social care services our service users are often feeling vulnerable and frightened and seek reassurance – sometimes putting even more pressure on staff who are struggling with their own feelings about change at work. If we can contribute to reducing the stress caused by frequent change, that in itself makes a contribution to improvement.

Change is driven from many different sources. Any one source may stimulate change in a particular area of activity, but there is often a wider impact. For example, if staff working hours are changed to provide services for longer hours this might represent a better service for service users. It may also cause a number of concerns. Staff may find the change in working hours disruptive to other aspects of their lives. Some staff may leave rather than comply with new require-ments. Arrangements for transport for staff to and from work may be disrupted. Transport patterns for service users may change. Costs of heating and lighting service delivery accommodation might increase to cover longer hours of use. There may be different catering requirements. Cleaning rotas may also have to change. More equip-ment and materials may be needed to cover longer hours of use. In service delivery, many aspects of provision are interconnected. The increased hours may not always represent an improvement to service users, particularly if what people really wanted was more choice rather than longer hours of access.

Health and social care services are essentially about people, both those who need to use services and those who provide services. People are sensitive to the impact of change and we have a partic-ular responsibility to take care over how we make changes in services that are intended to deliver care.

One of the reasons why change seems to be constant is that there are many potential stimuli for change and there are often several factors driving change at any one time. If change takes place in response to one stimulus, the impact is often spread across a range of issues. When change is taking place in response to a number of different driving factors, we may feel that the pace of change is running out of control.

The stimulus for change may come from inside an organisation or service area, but it is more usual for it to come from outside. Change initiated within an organisation or service area is often a response to a force outside the organisation that triggered the change.

CHANGE DRIVEN FROM THE EXTERNAL ENVIRONMENT

Most of the changes experienced in organisations are the result of factors in the external environment. For example, factors that have a significant impact on health and social care services include govern-ment policy and legislation, social change and technological change. Although the impact of change may be felt through internal changes, as in mergers or organisational restructuring, these are usually carried out in response to external pressures. One aspect of leadership is being able to look ahead and foresee some of the issues that your team will have to face in the future. One way of developing this foresight is to 'scan' the environment, to identify developments that will have an impact on your area of work.

A simple technique called 'STEEP analysis' can be used to help you to think about the external factors that might influence change in your organisation. STEEP stands for:

S sociological
T technological
E economic
E environmental
P political

You carry out a STEEP analysis by considering what factors in each of these categories are important in the external environment at the moment and what impact they are likely to have on your organisation or service area.

Example 8.1:   A STEEP analysis in health and care services

An organisation or agency providing services in health or social care might consider the following factors in making a STEEP analysis.

Sociological factors
Demographic and lifestyle factors can alter the nature of needs in a community and the expectations that individuals have of service provision. Each generation lives a little differently from that of their parents. Many sociological changes can be predicted when trends are identified. Central and local government provide statistical analysis of changes in social patterns. These statistics are usually widely available and are used by planners in health and care services to make long-term estimates of needs. For example, where the population of elderly people is increasing there will be an increase in demand for services for elderly people. Social factors that are likely to affect health and care services include demographic changes, patterns of work, patterns of consumption, gender roles and household structures.

The conditions in the locality served by your organisation will also be very important in assessing the impact of changes in sociological patterns. Families and groups with different backgrounds, traditions and values live in different ways. People living in different geographical areas face different conditions and respond to them in different ways. For example, services provided in inner-city areas are often very different from those provided in rural areas. Although it is important to consider national social trends, it is equally important to maintain a clear and critical perspective on what is relevant to your own situation.

Technological factors
Much of our activity in health and social care includes the use of technology and so is affected by technological developments. Communications

developments have brought increasing use of e-mail and mobile phones. Many organisations have difficulty in staying up to date with communications technology.

Service delivery is affected by developments in equipment and processes, but also by introductions in drugs and surgery that have enabled the pattern of provision to change so that some services can be delivered in non-traditional settings. New skills are often needed to make appropriate use of technological developments. Expectations of service users change as technology makes different methods of communication more convenient.

Use of the Internet for access to information has changed our ways of using records and libraries. Staff in health and care services have access to an increasing range of information through electronic libraries. Service users are able to access much of the information that is available to practitioners in health and social care. Service users expect us to make use of evidence in making decisions and databases of best practice models are increasingly available.

Economic factors
These factors include the general prosperity of the country and your neighbourhood, the rate of unemployment, areas of poverty, the level of inflation and exchange rates in relationships involving other countries and currencies.

The state of the economy affects the level of demand for goods and services, the prosperity of communities and the availability and cost of raw materials and of labour. The economy tends to move in cycles, but these are not easy to predict. All services, whether public services, private services or charity provision, are affected by changes in the economy.

Environmental factors
The sustainability of the natural environment has become a public concern. Organisations are increasingly expected to take care in how they dispose of or recycle waste, make use of energy, or impact upon their environment. For health and care organisations there are many concerns about how to manage waste of different types, how to manage energy and water, how to make efficient use of premises and how to address transport needs.

Political factors
Many aspects of health and social care are subject to legislation. New legal requirements emerge constantly as governments seek to improve health and social care, often through introduction of systems to set standards and to control or modify service provision. Legislation also affects service provision through legislation relating to employment, health and safety, pharmaceuticals, use of public funding and through related services including education and housing. Political factors also influence the ways in which services are offered and the degree of regulation controlling the provision, including regulation of staff and professions and regulation of buildings and equipment.

The STEEP framework provides a useful structure for identifying the key factors that you can expect to have an impact on your organisation or service area in the near future. There is a degree of overlap in the categories, but this is not important if you use the model to help you to think about the environmental factors that might affect your area of work.

ACTIVITY 8.2

Allow 10 minutes.

Look back through the description of each of the STEEP factors and consider how each of these might affect your area of work during the next year or so. Focus on issues that you expect that your team will have to respond to in some way. Make a note of the five most significant issues:

1 _____

2 _____

3 _____

4 _____

5 _____

These issues are the ones that could provide opportunities for you to take a leadership role. Consider how your team might prepare to respond to one or two of the issues and discuss it with your colleagues. If you find that others support your ideas, think about how you might gain support from senior colleagues to take your ideas forward.

WHAT CHOICE DO WE HAVE?

As we have said, people have different views of change. Those who dislike change of any sort may put up barriers to try to prevent, or at least to delay, change. Those who welcome change may try to initiate it and seek opportunities to be involved in introducing changes. It is possible that our attitudes towards change are shaped, to some extent, by the degree of involvement we have in planning and structuring the change.

Most of the work in health and social care organisations is carried out in teams. These teams often have a choice about how they plan and carry out their activities. Teams can also choose how to work in settings where change is likely to be frequent. There are two choices, to be reactive to change or to be proactive. Teams that are reactive do not try to foresee changes and may try to ignore the need to change until they are forced to react, to respond only when absolutely necessary. Teams that are proactive look ahead and plan how to change the ways in which they do things so that they keep abreast of changing needs. The reactive response often leads to a rather jerky working life in which there are longish periods of stability until the need to change is so great that not only must change be made but it has to be significant change. The proactive response often provides a way of working that accommodates continuous minor change, incremental change, as part of normal work.

Proactive response to change is only possible when members of the team notice the need to change and are able to share this awareness with other members of the team. This may lead to suggestions of ways in which the team might react. Leadership is essential in raising awareness of the need to change and in shaping a proactive response. This type of leadership may come from anyone in a team.

CHANGE DRIVEN FROM WITHIN THE ORGANISATION

Sometimes it seems as though change is being driven from within an organisation. For example, the finance department might announce that they would like to open consultation about introducing a new budgeting system. If you are responsible for a budget, you may be invited to meetings or interviewed about the way in which you find the current budgeting processes useful or unhelpful. The proposals for changing the system may come directly from the finance department, but something will have triggered the idea. It might have been triggered by concern about overspending in some areas of work that might be addressed by improving the ways in which budgets are developed. It might also have been triggered by external criticism of lack of control of overspending. The overspending might have arisen because of inaccurate forecasts of service needs. This might have arisen because the organisation had been provided with poor information by other agencies.

It is sometimes difficult to determine whether drivers for change arise externally or internally, but if an organisation is not aware of developments in its environment it will soon be seen as out of touch and out of date. You may think that it's not so bad to be a little old-fashioned, but whether organisations are financed by public or private money, those who invest in them will be expecting resources to be used efficiently and effectively. They expect that the finance available will be used to best effect in providing high-quality services.

When you scan the environment to consider what is driving change, you will probably be aware of different pressures impacting on different areas of the work of your organisation. It is quite likely that a finance department might be the first to respond to pressure related to use of funding, or a human resource department to be the first to respond to staffing shortages. It is unlikely, however, that change driven by any department could be initiated without the involvement of all other parts of the organisation. Systems are connected to each other and operate alongside each other to support the work of the organisation. An approach to change that proposed change to only one system or a part of a system would usually indicate that the impact on other systems had not been considered. This is why an approach that takes all of the systems into consideration, a whole systems approach, is usually advised. An approach that takes a whole systems overview will consider the impact of change on the whole organisation. Proposed benefits in one area of work can possibly be aligned to produce wider benefits or, at least, to avoid causing new problems in one area to achieve a possible benefit in another.

TYPES OF CHANGE

Different types of change have different characteristics and different implications for the people and organisations involved.

- *Incremental change* – This is continuous and can become a way of working that enables a team or organisation to keep up with changes in the demands made of it. This can arise from a concern for continuous improvement and is often welcomed by people who value reflective practice as continuous personal development. The success of incremental change depends on the skills of those involved in accurately predicting the type and scale of change that is required in order to maintain services that respond to all the demands made of them.
- *Step change* – This is change that is significant and provides a leap from one position to another. This is the type of change that affects many aspects of an organisation, because in making one significant change in one area of work there will usually be a knock-on effect that influences many other aspects of work. An example of a step change is when a completely new service is introduced or a service discontinued, or when a service is moved to a new location.
- *Transformational change* – This is more significant than a step change because it creates a new condition, a new identity. The change is profound for all those associated in transformational change because everyone has to change themselves in order to relate to the new identity. For example, when two organisations that have different staff and different areas of expertise merge to enable more cost-effective service provision in a geographical area, staff and service users have to develop a new understanding of the new organisation.

The scale of change is also important in considering the impact that it is likely to have on the people involved. Very large-scale change is usually directed from the highest levels of an organisation because of the complexity of linking multiple areas of services. Small-scale changes can take place in any area of work, although it may be necessary to seek approval, particularly if there will be changes to the way in which the area of work interacts with collaborating service areas.

The word '*transformational*' is increasingly used to indicate change that makes a significant difference, transforms a situation. '*Transactional*' is used, sometimes in rather a derogatory way, to mean management through individual transactions rather than an holistic approach. '*Transcendent*' is also sometimes used to talk about a visionary idea that rises above usual expectations.

WORKING IN COMPLEX SYSTEMS

Health and social care settings are complex because of the number of interactions that are necessary in order to deliver the various aspects of a service. Each service area has many systems that enable consistent delivery of that area of work. As each of these areas of work experiences change, these systems have to change. Changes happen at different rates and it is often necessary to continue to run old systems until the new ones are proven consistent enough to replace the old. This can mean that in any area of work there are both new and old systems running alongside each other, each trying to make appropriate links with systems in other areas of work to enable provision of linked services.

The attempt to provide 'joined-up' services is often hindered by the difficulties of linking so many elements that are each undergoing their own sets of changes. Not only do the systems each change at different speeds, but considerable adaptation is taking place as people become aware of the new approaches replacing the old. Where staff in health and social care are focused on the experience of the service user or patient, the difficulties of constant change can be modified and service users can be offered the best options available. The complexity of change in these closely interlinked services can be both confusing and frightening for service users, but local leaders can recognise the problems that service users might face during periods of change and can provide guidance to help people to find a pathway through the apparent chaos.

MODELS OF CHANGE

The ideas we have discussed about scanning the external environment to develop foresight about drivers for change are well known but not always put into practice. It is sometimes said that change is easy to discuss in terms of models and ideas, but very much more difficult to understand in practice. One of the reasons for this is that we can consider ideas and change models without these having very much impact on our feelings or our emotions. Once a change becomes something we are living and not simply discussing, we experience it through all of our senses and responses. This is much more complicated than discussing possibilities. Models of change processes give us a sense of order and control that help us to think about aspects of change without dwelling too much on the potential difficulties.

You might be suspecting by now that too much emphasis is being put on how people feel and that change might be more easily accomplished by simply issuing orders, and staff who don't like the changes will conform or leave. There is a model (Gleicher, 1986) that sets out the conditions for successful change in the form of a pseudo-mathematical equation:

If A = the individual's or group's level of dissatisfaction with things
as they are now;
and B = the individual's or group's shared vision of a better future;
and C = the existence of an acceptable, safe first step;
and D = the costs to the individual or group;
then change is unlikely unless:
A + B + C is greater than D.

The assumption in this model is that people are not likely to be interested in change unless they see the benefits as outweighing the costs.
All of the conditions described here are ones that people perceive and
perceptions can be influenced and changed. You might feel very
dissatisfied with something that others seem not to be worried about.
If people are comfortable with how things are, they are unlikely to
want change or support attempts to make changes. If people don't
see the advantages of a proposal, they will be unlikely to support it
– so a vision has to be clear and fairly unambiguous to attract
support. If the vision appears to threaten individuals, they will be
very unlikely to offer support and may become active in trying to
prevent change. If people accept that change is necessary but are
worried about the scale of change and the implications for themselves
or their work, a limited change may offer a way forward. A safe first
step might provide reassurance and encouragement to consider
further developments.

Perhaps the most simple model describing the process of change is
the idea that change is about moving from A to B. If our current state
is A and the new, desired state is B, change is what needs to happen
to move from A to B. This model depends on clarity about what we
mean by A (not easy to define in complex settings with many inter-
locking systems) and what we mean by B (also not always easy to
define). A very simple change might be visualised using this model
and the steps from A to B identified. The danger with such a linear
model is that many of the contextual implications would be ignored.

Example 8.2: Lewin's three-stage model of change

One model of change has been enduring in helping people to think about
change, the idea proposed by Lewin (1947) that there are three stages in
any change:

■ unfreezing;
■ moving;
■ re-freezing.

The unfreezing stage is when people begin to accept that there is a need for
change. The second stage of moving is when it is possible to make changes.
The third stage of re-freezing is when the change is consolidated and the
changed state becomes the new normal state.

This simple image reminds us of the need to allow time for people to come to terms with the possibility of change. This may include recognising past achievements that served the organisation well but are no longer suitable for new conditions. Sometimes an event shocks people into realising that change is not only inevitable but also necessary. For example, a report into the events that contributed to a scandal or tragedy in a health or social care setting can stimulate staff and service users into demanding change to prevent similar events in future. At other times people may need to be involved in consideration of whether change is necessary. For example, when new legislation is introduced that requires all organisations to provide particular types of access or services for disabled people, most organisations need to review the extent to which they currently meet the requirements and plan changes to ensure that they comply. It is much easier to engage people in making changes once they are committed to the proposal that change must happen.

The image of being able to make changes when the organisation is unfrozen suggests that everything has to loosen a little to accommodate change. This can be a helpful reminder that change can rarely be accomplished in one area without impact on at least the immediately adjacent areas of work. This image of unfreezing can also remind us that there is possibly a limited time in which everything can be kept flexible enough to change. It might be important to be well prepared so that plans can be implemented quickly and decisively.

The re-freezing stage is one in which the change is confirmed and becomes the new way of doing things. This is not such an easy image to apply now that we are aware of the constancy and frequency of change. It does remind us, however, that we need to establish new ways of working so that they do become the accepted processes if the change is to stick and people will not be tempted to revert to former ways of working.

Lewin's model of change is more holistic than a simple A to B model, but it also has limitations in its focus on time-scales. It seems to suggest that everything that needs to be changed can be accomplished more or less at the same time, so that it can all be re-frozen into the new ways of working. This is unlikely in complex settings where it will usually be necessary to keep systems working while change is carried out, so change will often have to be accomplished alongside existing work.

A systems view of change offers a model that focuses on the work of the organisation or service area in its context. An example of a systems model of service change is given in Example 8.3 and Figure 8.1.

Example 8.3:   A systems model of service change

This model is about how resources are transformed into the service as it is delivered to service users. The box on the left represents the inputs, including the resources that are available to produce and provide the service. The box in the middle represents the transformation of these basic resources that is necessary to turn them into a service. The box on the right represents outputs of all of the activity in the central box, the results of providing the service.

The 'inputs' include the people who require the service, the resources that are used to provide the service and the environment that impacts on provision of the service. The people who become the service users bring their own needs but also some resources, both physical and in the form of their attitudes and abilities available to support themselves. The resources available to provide the service include staff and funding for materials, equipment and the service environment. The wider environment includes the local community, the social, technological, economic, environmental and political conditions and the history of the organisation or service.

This systems model does not show how the transformation takes place, but the interactions that are necessary to produce the service. Thus the model might be seen not as a model of one single change, but as a model of the continuous change activity involved in service delivery. Our day-to-day work involves making changes as we use our thinking and actions as people to work with equipment, materials, premises, time and other resources to produce health and care services. An implicit assumption of continuous change is inevitable in such a range of interactions because these are human activities and unlikely to ever be repeated in exactly the same way each time they are enacted.

We should notice that the inputs and outputs might also change and that either of these changes would produce a need to do things differently in the central box. If the resources were increased or became more constrained, there would be implications for the activities in the transformation and for the eventual outputs. If the requirements of the outputs change, then both inputs and activities may have to change to meet the new requirements.

This model has been shown as representing a single service, but any service has a number of systems that contribute to making it work. There are formal systems that deal with employment of staff, the human resource or personnel systems. There are financial systems that deal with obtaining money from a variety of sources, planning use of that money to obtain physical resources and to pay staff, accounting for the use of the money and reporting on what has been achieved with the funding provided. There will be systems that organise how service users receive the service, including how they are informed, registered, given appointments and how the service is delivered to each individual user. Other systems deal with premises, health and safety issues, cleaning, catering, transport and other things. Most of these examples are of formal systems that have been regularised into routine ways of working. There are also informal systems that staff develop to make things work in each particular setting. These include arrangements that individuals make as ways of working with each other, favours that one person regularly offers others, patterns of work that include social processes and traditions that have developed. In considering change, the informal processes that are part of the culture of an organisation can be overlooked but might be more resistant to change than the formal structures because the informal ways of working are often perceived to be 'owned' by staff rather than by the organisation.

This is a systems model of change because it gives an overview that demonstrates that transformation is carried out through interaction of a number of systems.

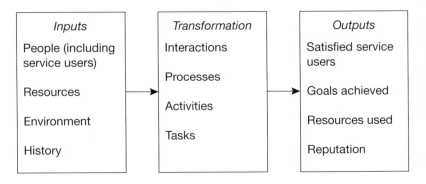

Figure 8.1   A systems model of service change

LEADING TRANSFORMATIONAL CHANGE

Models of change give us some indication of the sorts of actions that are needed if we are to be proactive in responding to signs that change is needed. If we are not proactive, we will find ourselves reacting to the pressures as they build up. This may leave us little time to think or plan how we would like to respond. A reactive approach to change is risky because it implies not doing anything until it is unavoidable and, perhaps, then doing only the minimum to respond to the immediate pressure. If we are forced into a series of reactive responses, we may soon find ourselves out of control with unplanned changes in a number of areas and with no mechanisms to link processes and systems together again. Leadership is needed to develop a proactive response to pressure to change. Leadership is needed to develop and keep a clear sense of direction, to find pathways and to show how the path can be followed.

The systems model identifies the arena in which transformation takes place and demonstrates the dynamic relationship between inputs, transformational systems and outputs. We might develop this model by adding the process cycle of leadership that was introduced in Chapter 1 (Figure 1.2) to produce a model of transformational leadership in service development (Figure 8.2).

In the transformation process we can no longer think of leadership as an individual pursuit. It is a group process in which there is not a single inspirational person 'at the top', but individuals within groups who influence attitudes and inspiration at all levels of the organisation. When we consider the number of systems that contribute to the transformation of inputs to a service into delivery of that service, we can see the extent to which leadership will be needed to stimulate and progress any change. We can apply the process model of leading change to the transformation 'box' of the

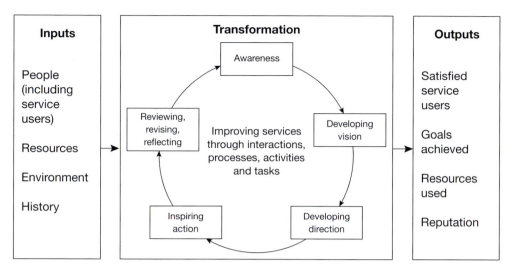

Figure 8.2   Leading transformational change

systems diagram to probe more deeply into the implications of making change in a complex service area.

The first stage of being aware involves having an overview of the environment and the pressures for change, together with an understanding of the ways in which your organisation currently converts its resources (inputs) into service delivery (outputs). It also implies understanding of pressures to make changes that will represent improvements in the service. The next stage, developing vision, focuses on developing a picture of what a better service might be like. We consider this in more detail in Chapter 10. Developing direction involves examining the inputs, transformation processes and outputs to develop steps and pathways that will progress the changes that are necessary to achieve the vision. This is discussed more fully in Chapter 11. Once the direction has been agreed, the focus moves to inspiring action. If the processes of developing vision and direction have been collaborative, engagement in the process will often generate enthusiasm for action. If, however, the process has been slow or interrupted, it may be necessary to re-energise people to inspire them to act. Chapter 12 explores ways in which we might lead and contribute to this stage in the change process. Once some progress has been made, reviewing and revision can begin. Reflection is beneficial throughout the change process, but at this stage we can consider the extent to which the whole process has been successful in moving towards achieving the vision. This is discussed in Chapter 13.

In this chapter we have considered the importance of being aware of the pressures that stimulate change and the potential impact of change on your organisation or service area and the people who interact there. We concluded by bringing these issues together in a model of the process of leading change to transform an organisation or service area. The stages in the process are explored in the following chapters.

CHAPTER 9

FINDING A FOCUS

Being aware is only the beginning of the process of focusing on what changes would make a significant difference. Our own perceptions of a situation are limited, but we rarely realise our own limitations until we listen carefully to opinions offered by other people. Perceptions and opinions are slippery things, although very important ones in shaping our beliefs and actions. We usually want to find out whether there is any less emotive evidence relating to a situation before we feel confident in making a judgement about how to respond. In this chapter we review some of the ways in which we might find out more and develop a richer understanding of a situation or problem. We also consider how we might ensure that any change we propose presents the possibility of improvement rather than simply something different.

MAKING AN IMPROVEMENT

Change does not automatically lead to improvement. The idea of improvement is complex, as what represents improvement to one person or group may be seen as a loss or cost to others. Those who doubt that improvement will result from the proposal or those who see undesirable consequences often challenge proposals of improvement. We should remember that 'quality is in the eye of the beholder'.

Sometimes it is easy to gain agreement that things are not working as well as we would like them to be working, but it is not as easy to agree what might be done to improve things. The process of identifying areas for improvement needs some thought and planning. We need to agree about what needs improvement and what contributary factors should be considered, what we need to do to make the improvement and what the result of the improvement will be. In systems thinking terms, this means considering the inputs, the outputs and the transformation processes.

It might seem logical to think first about how the outputs could be improved. This might be the best starting position if there is a widely agreed need to make an improvement in the outputs. This situation might arise when standards have to be improved or when more has to be achieved with little increase in the resource inputs. Sometimes, however, change in the inputs brings pressure to change the transformational processes if the outputs are not to be reduced in quality or quantity. In health and care services, change in the transformational processes can also lead to a need for wider change. For example, a treatment procedure may be changed in response to evidence that one procedure is much more effective than others in current use. There will be pressure for all services to use the most effective procedure instead of less effective ones. A change in the way things are done for one procedure will usually have a number of implications for other aspects of the area of work. For example, the number of staff who are needed to engage with service users might change and bring differences in appointments and schedules, staffing needs and accommodation needs for service users. This will, in turn, bring associated differences in requirements from all the supporting administrative and facilities services. In complex services, any change may have multiple implications.

Leaders and change agents need to retain personal credibility if they are to gain the trust and support of others to progress change. It is wise to invest time and energy to develop understanding of a situation in the early stages of your awareness of the need for change. There are various ways in which you might do this. We will consider several different approaches that can be used separately or together, depending on the nature and scale of possible change. As a 'rule of thumb', the scale of change is one of the key issues in considering how much time and energy to invest in developing a shared understanding of the issues. The greater the scale, the more potential there is for misunderstanding.

We can assess the scale of the potential change using a simple model that is usually called 'messes and difficulties' (see Example 9.1 and Figure 9.1).

Example 9.1:   Messes and difficulties

One way to consider different types of change is to separate problems that are fairly easy to understand, where the change needed to solve the problem is fairly clear, from changes that are complex and wide-ranging. A technique that will help you to do this separates problem areas into 'messes' and 'difficulties'.

A *difficulty* is limited and can be treated as a project with a clear purpose, time-scale and resource needs. A *mess* is much more difficult to understand and needs time and energy invested to investigate it before any action can be taken to solve the problem or improve the situation. In a mess the problem might not even be evident, as the symptoms are usually recognised before the roots of the problem are understood. Sorting problems into messes and difficulties has the benefit of differentiating those problems that can be addressed by a project with a clear purpose that is likely to bring a successful change from the messy problem areas that have much wider-ranging implications and which will need a different approach.

Difficulties and messes can be identified by their characteristics.

Figure 9.1 shows a difficulty as a boundaried shape around a problem and a mess as a shape with a dotted boundary. In each case there are spokes from the 'problem' at the centre with the following characteristics:

Messes – unbounded problems – have the following characteristics:

- Bigger
- Unlimited people involved
- Unbounded
- Long time-scale
- Wide implications
- Uncertain problem
- No clear solution
- Don't know what needs to be known
- Can't disentangle from context
- Unclear priorities

Difficulties – bounded problems – have the following characteristics:

- Smaller
- Limited number of people involved
- Bounded
- Short time-scale
- Limited implications
- Certain problem
- Know a likely solution
- Know what needs to be known
- Can treat as a separate matter
- Clear priorities

You can use these characteristics to help to decide whether the situation that you face is a difficulty (in which case it might be handled as a limited project) or a mess, which will need much wider involvement to understand and address. There are tried and tested approaches to the management of projects and the results are likely to be successful if those working on the project organise and manage their work effectively. For more information and help in managing projects in health and social care settings you may like to consult Martin (2002). If you have enjoyed using this approach to sorting out the problems that can be addressed in a straightforward way from the problems that will take much more time and trouble, you might enjoy learning more about a systems approach to change introduced in Carter et al. (1984).

Messes are much more complex and will take time to understand before a diagnosis can be made and options for change considered. Change in unbounded areas of complex settings is complicated and often has numerous implications, but there are techniques and approaches that can help at all stages of understanding and making change.

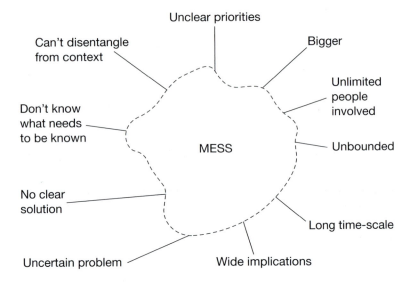

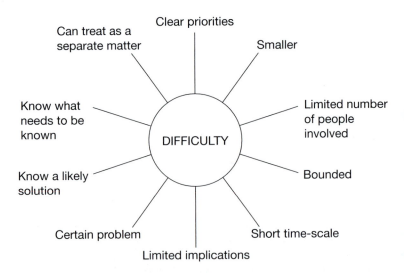

Figure 9.1   Messes and difficulties

In most areas of work there are a range of problems, some of which can be identified as 'difficulties' and some of which are definitely 'messes'. You can identify a difficulty by considering the character-istics. For example, you might be considering change in the way details of service users are collected on initial registration. If the numbers of staff using these details are small, if the numbers of staff taking the details are restricted and if the numbers of service users are not particularly large, you might have a difficulty rather than a problem. If the area in which you are considering making a change does not link closely with others who rely on the records in the form they are currently in, you may have a boundary around the problem area that would enable you to treat it as a difficulty. If some action needs to be taken quickly and the implications for other people and other areas of work are very limited, this may be straightforward to address. If you are certain about what is causing the problem and if there is already some agreement about what might be done to solve the problem, you might be able to treat this as a separate and limited change. You might already have all the information that is necessary to plan the change and you might have already identified the priorities. A limited change of this nature can be treated as a 'difficulty' and managed as a project. If the implications are wider, you will need to approach the situation as a 'mess'.

GETTING INTO A MESS

Once you have decided that you are trying to understand a 'mess' and that you cannot treat it as a limited difficulty, you will need to take an approach that unravels some of the issues that contribute to the complexity. One approach that can explore the dynamic relationships in a situation is the rich picture (see Example 9.2).

Example 9.2:   A rich picture

A 'rich picture' is a drawing that gives a rich description of a situation. It can be drawn by an individual or a group. If drawn by an individual, it will show one perspective on the situation, but if drawn by a group it may capture a wider perspective or an agreed overview.

The picture is intended to capture the complexity of a situation, showing all of the groups and individuals involved and indicating some of the types of communications between them, including collaboration and conflicts. It would usually show something of the different locations involved and any connections between them, perhaps showing how the inputs and outputs relate and what transformations take place. The complications are often in the transforming areas and these may have additional information displayed as 'thought' or 'speech bubbles'. A rich picture (see Figure 9.2) is usually drawn using pictures, symbols and connecting lines. If it is drawn by a group, it attempts to capture a discussion about the relationships and difficulties within the situation. An individual can only capture her or his own view, but this can then provide material for a discussion with others.

This approach is often used as a first step in beginning to understand the complexities in a situation and the technique is derived from systems thinking, from Checkland (1981).

Rich pictures capture some of the emotional aspects of a situation and so are often provocative when used to stimulate group discussion. One of the main uses of a rich picture is to identify where there are blockages or problems in the sequences that represent the transformative activities, the activities that are the tasks of the organisation and that produce its outcomes.

It is usually helpful to ask the person or people who drew the picture to explain the features. If you have drawn the picture and will analyse it yourself, it is still helpful to look through it and identify the main issues and themes that it represents.

In this picture the perspective is one taken by a person who works on a reception desk in a small primary care practice. She explains the picture:

> There are two doctors and one nurse who have appointments to see patients. The patients come to the practice, tell us they're here and then wait for their appointment. The doctors and nurse expect us (there are two part-time receptionists) to bring the patient records for each appointment and also to show the patients to the appropriate rooms.
>
> There are never enough times for appointments and patients can become angry and anxious when they want to see a doctor urgently. The phones never stop ringing, not just for appointments but with all sorts of questions. All the calls from the hospital, from Social Services and from the local agencies come through reception and the Practice Manager is usually too busy to answer, so we have to take messages. The Practice Manager is new to the job and just seems to worry about numbers and money all the time. One of the doctors is very difficult to deal with and always seems to be causing offence. The other is a close friend of the Practice Nurse, so they get on well. The doctors and nurse are always making different arrangements among themselves and they don't tell us what's happening. So then they blame us when things go wrong. We always seem to be sitting under a big black cloud!
>
> Records are a real problem. There is never time to file them at the end of the day, so we try to do that in between other things – but since we're busy all the time it doesn't often get done properly. That means that we often can't find a person's records when they're needed, so everyone gets cross. But we always have to deal with the person who's in front of us before we deal with the paper. We're supposed to be putting the records onto a computerised system, but I can't see how that will ever happen.
>
> It is discussed in meetings sometimes, but everyone seems to have different ideas about what the problems are in this practice and what we might do about them. We both feel like leaving because it all seems impossible to sort out.

'At the heart of a learning organization is a shift of mind – from seeing ourselves as separate from the world to connected to the world, from seeing problems as caused by someone or something "out there" to seeing how our own actions create the problems we experience. A learning organization is a place where people are continually discovering how they create their reality. And how they can change it.'
(Senge, 1990, pp. 12–13)

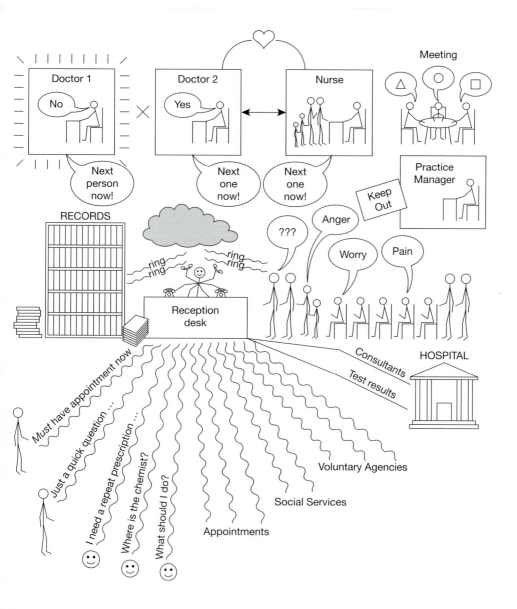

Figure 9.2   Rich picture of being on reception in a primary care practice

ACTIVITY 9.1

Allow 10 minutes.

How would you help this receptionist to analyse this situation? First of all, from the rich picture in Figure 9.2, what are the inputs and how do they get transformed into the outputs?

Inputs	Transformation	Outputs
_____	_____	_____
_____	_____	_____
_____	_____	_____
_____	_____	_____
_____	_____	_____

The inputs you might have identified include people wanting an appointment with a doctor or nurse, information (in the form of telephone messages, test results, hospital appointments, financial information), whatever the doctors and nurses need as equipment and materials. The transformation includes doctors and nurses talking to, examining and possibly treating patients, information being recorded, used and filed and questions being answered. The outputs are people who have had appointments with doctors and the nurse, some of whom need to make further appointments. There are also information outputs that relate to individual patients and, presumably, overall records of the activity levels of the practice for funding purposes.

You might have also noted the tensions and frustration indicated in the picture. Now try to identify the main things that are causing tension.

_____

_____

_____

_____

_____

One of the main causes of tension is that the reception desk is the centre of activity in the practice. You might wonder if it only looks like that because of the perception of the person who drew the picture. It does appear, however, that all the communications that come into and go out of the practice pass through the reception staff. With only two people there and possibly only one at a time working at the reception desk, this does look like a bottleneck. The big black cloud is important to notice too – the receptionists seem to feel strong disapproval and there is no evidence that they are getting support from anywhere. Meetings don't seem to offer any shared communication. The Practice Manager's door seems to be firmly shut. The records system is still paper-based and records are not always available when they are needed. The patients seem to be waiting a lot in long queues and some are anxious, some angry.

A number of issues here offer opportunities for improvement. You may already be able to suggest some actions that might make an immediate improvement. For example, you might be thinking that the Practice Manager could make all the communications with the hospital, Social Services and other agencies to reduce the range of contacts dealt with at reception. This suggestion might be welcomed by the receptionists, but might be rejected by the Practice Manager, who is unlikely to see any personal benefits in taking on additional work. You might have thought that the doctors and nurse could come into the waiting area and ask for their next patient instead of involving reception. Again, they might not welcome this activity, particularly if there are frustrated and angry people there who might accost them. Another idea might be to set up modernisation of the records system as a project. This would have to be funded and those using the system would need to find time for training, but patients increasingly expect records to be kept accurately and to be available when needed.

A rich picture can be used, as we have in this activity, to indicate some areas for potential change. They can also be further analysed to enable diagnosis of particular problem areas. The best people to do this diagnosis are those who are closely involved in the situation because they understand different aspects of the complexity. If, however, everyone is to be involved, both the drawing of the picture and the analysis have to be carefully facilitated so that individuals do not feel that they can be identified as the ones to blame for failure. This can be difficult when individuals hold key roles, but discussion of the constraints governing particular roles rather than the ways in which different personalities behave can make discussion possible and fruitful.

Ideally, analysis of a rich picture will identify which specific systems within the situation are causing difficulties. Those analysing the picture will, ideally, be able to say what they would like to change. At this stage it should be possible to describe in words which key systems need to be changed. Once this has been achieved, the diagnosis is complete and it is possible to work out how the picture would look if things were all working perfectly (the vision) and how to make these changes (the direction). We will return to these further stages in systems thinking in Chapters 10 and 11.

ASKING QUESTIONS

Another way to identify what needs to change is to ask people. If, however, we simply ask what should change to make an improvement, there is a danger that we will collect many contradictory ideas without identifying focal areas for change. People will have different views of a situation and will make different interpretations. To gain a broad perspective, it will be necessary to question people who are likely to hold different views. One way of exploring the potential for change in an area of work is to focus on the outcomes. Instead of asking what is going wrong, ask individuals what better outcomes would look like. Sometimes people will offer opinions about how better outcomes might be achieved, often thinking that more resources or time would improve results, but try to focus on what better results would be like. Sometimes a group of people from one area of work can do this together, to develop a description that they agree would be an improvement in the results of their work.

Another way to approach this type of questioning is to ask what would make a person proud of their work. For example, you might set a scenario by asking people to think about how the work that they do might be reported in the press in a year's time. They have been extraordinarily successful and their results have attracted wide attention. Ask them to list the main points that would be reported – what would this success be like?

If you are more comfortable with asking very open questions, you might interview a range of individuals who each hold a different view on an area of work, perhaps because of their roles in the setting. You might start your questions by asking a person to tell you what they think is a successful outcome from their area of work. You can encourage them to give you as much description as possible by asking, when they seem to have finished, 'Can you tell me any more?' This question can be asked until no more ideas are offered. Sometimes probing in this way can reveal much more about what people believe to be excellent outcomes. This type of questioning can sometimes lead to limited answers if people feel exhausted and have been struggling to work without adequate resources. It is most successful when people are able to imagine a better future.

Another area that can sometimes be approached well through direct questioning is that of values underlying an area of work. Your initial question might be, 'What values are important to you in your work?' and you might then follow this by probing, asking if they can tell you more. You may find that there is considerable consistency in the values expressed and this may provide a focal area if people do not think that their values are being demonstrated in their current ways of working.

History might also provide a way to identify a focus for change. People are often able to talk about work that they were proud of in the past. You might ask about past work and ask what was good about it, why they still feel proud of it. Then ask what would make them proud of their current work. This can be a helpful approach if people feel that there has been a deterioration in performance or outcomes but find it difficult to be specific about what is different. The perception is often that more has to be done with fewer resources and with less time, and questions that contrast the past with the present can help to show whether the source of dissatisfaction is more in the working processes or in the results of that work.

It is important to find a focus that many people are concerned about so that attempts to make changes will be supported. It is not possible to develop a vision of a future that will inspire people to make changes unless they care enough about the possibility and believe that there is some hope of making improvements. Spending some time in exploring the focal areas can raise awareness and begin to awaken the interest that will be needed to gain momentum to create change.

CHAPTER 10

DEVELOPING VISION

Many people are uneasy with the idea of developing a vision. The word implies something creative, perhaps mystical, idealistic or romantic and certainly rather unusual. A vision is an idea, but one that can be described in a way that enables it to be shared with others. This chapter begins by discussing the nature of vision, both as a way of seeing ideas and as something that can be deliberately constructed.

We consider some of the ways in which you can develop and capture a vision. Different approaches will attract different people. Some are comfortable with allowing imagination to range freely and others are much more comfortable with approaches that build on more concrete foundations. Similarly, if a vision is to be widely shared, different approaches will have to be taken to communicating the ideas and building the vision in a way that is meaningful to all those involved.

Collaboration in developing vision is very important to gain shared commitment, but in complex settings people often have very different ideas about priorities. This can lead to development of a number of conflicting visions. These need to be reconciled if people are to be able to work together towards one shared vision of a desirable future. Commitment to a vision is an essential step before commitment to a direction can be developed.

THE NATURE OF VISION

Vision, in the context of change, is an idea about the future. We all have such ideas, all of the time. If someone asks you what you want, you might give a very practical reply or you might give a reply that you think is exaggerated and fanciful, something that could never happen. Both are visions. Visions are ordinary experiences and influence our everyday decisions.

Visions can also be ideas that provide hope. Someone who is lost in a desert and who has been struggling to progress without water might see a vision of an oasis and gain the strength from that hope to go a little further. Visions can inspire us to make an extra effort.

Visions can provide ideas that describe a future that looks attractive to us, a dream of what might be. As we each have different hopes, fears and concerns, shared visions might have multiple facets that offer different types of attractions to different people. When a vision is of a future that will be shared by many different people, it is advisable to develop that vision with wide involvement so that the variety of interests can be included in thinking about the future.

Visions can be powerful because they can interact with our hopes and fears, with our values and with our need to see some continuity into the future. This is why visions are so important as part of leading change. A clear and shared vision of a better future is very inspiring and motivating. If the vision is accompanied by plans for progress that appear to be achievable, people will often want to put energy into making the vision a reality. Leading includes understanding the value of vision and being able to develop vision both as an individual and with your group.

Vision is associated with creativity because creating a vision involves creating something that did not exist before or, maybe, making something visible that was not evident before. People sometimes think that they are not creative. Let us consider what we understand by creativity.

ACTIVITY 10.1

Allow 5 minutes.

Where do ideas come from? Where do your ideas come from? Make a list:

_____

_____

_____

_____

_____

Were you able to identify some of the sources of your own ideas? You might have thought that your ideas often come from hearing or reading about what other people think. Sometimes we pick up an idea and can use it directly, but often we shape it and apply it to our own circumstances. Sometimes an idea might seem to come out of nowhere, just appearing as an inspiration. At other times we might be aware of putting two ideas together and coming up with something rather unexpected. Some people do this deliberately as a way of provoking more unusual ideas. People who think laterally, linking ideas from different areas of their perception and experience, often find that linked ideas produce surprises. Often people who are able to use different approaches to developing new ideas are thought to be creative people.

'I have a dream . . .'

There is no one way of developing ideas, dreams or visions. There are, however, some conditions in which creativity flourishes and conditions that dampen or prevent creative thinking. Creativity can blossom if it is nurtured. Rather than focusing on how to provoke creativity, simply providing the conditions in which it can grow naturally will usually produce it.

WHAT STOPS US FROM BEING CREATIVE?

Constant pressure to carry out tasks and produce results in limited time drives out creativity because we need space to consider doing things differently. Repeating activities in the same way ensures that similar results will usually be obtained and no-one will be at risk of being blamed for failure to follow procedures. Several issues are raised here.

1 Regulating activity through inflexible processes and procedures can lead to emphasis on repetitive behaviour without consideration of whether it continues to be the best way of doing things. There are advantages in having protocols where these are the currently agreed best practice in particular circumstances, but flexibility is often also important. Guidelines can be more helpful than regulations when there is an option. Organisations that attempt to regularise many of their processes and procedures risk driving creativity away. This may seem a good thing at the time that a process is regulated, but conditions change and any process is at risk of failing to meet current demands if it is constrained by outdated regulation.
2 Once processes, procedures and protocols become the prescribed ways of doing things, people are expected to conform or face some form of punishment. This reduces a sense of responsibility for achieving good results and puts an emphasis on doing what is required regardless of the quality of the result.
3 Regulation of processes brings a value to conformity rather than collaboration to achieve a purpose. Those who conform are valued above those who want to do better. A 'blame' culture can develop in which there is an expectation that someone will be blamed if anything goes wrong.

4 Continuous development is impossible if behaviour is too tightly constrained by regulation of processes.

5 Critical reflective practitioners have little opportunity to develop in settings that are too tightly regulated. Lack of these people reduces an organisations's ability to respond in positive ways to pressure to change.

Concern about safe and efficient practice often drives pressure to regulate. The advantages of regulation appear to offer reassurance that standards can be maintained. The disadvantages in terms of reducing the ability of staff to be innovative and to take responsibility for their actions are rarely considered. Introduction of regimes of regulation and inspection to ensure conformity can drive out the creativity that is needed to provide innovative responses to future conditions.

Associated with the restrictions that highly regulated situations can bring are cultural conditions that prevent any challenge to the existing regime. An example in health and care services can be found in some professions where there are many barriers that make it difficult to consider change. To some extent this can be the result of developing regulation that was, perhaps, necessary to develop and establish standards. Professional education also often emphasises a particular way of thinking and acting that is regarded as 'professional' and which those joining the profession are expected to emulate. This makes it very difficult for those in the profession or outside it to challenge what is considered to be the professional model. This is not to suggest that professions are bad for health and care services, but that regulation and suppression of challenge cannot prepare people to think and act in new and different ways when conditions change.

Professions also provide some potential answers to this dilemma. Principles and values that underpin behaviour provide a basis for judgement. Professional judgement based on an understanding of principles and values can be flexible to accommodate differences in circumstances and people. Principles and values can be discussed and can become a foundation for inter-professional working. New ways of doing things can be developed in teams of mixed professions and disciplines. But only if time and space and loose enough regulation permit.

Another barrier to creativity is lack of hope. When people are exhausted and can see no possibility of a better future, they struggle to keep going and lack the energy to become inspired or to participate in creating a vision. They may even fear any approach that might ask a little more of them if they are already giving as much as they can.

'Forces that threaten to negate life must be challenged by courage, which is the power of life to affirm itself in spite of life's ambiguities. This requires the exercise of a creative will that enables us to hew out a stone of hope from a mountain of despair.' (Rev. Martin Luther King, Jr.)

WHAT HELPS US TO BE CREATIVE?

Having considered the depressing circumstances in which creativity is difficult, there is good news about what helps us to be creative. It is more about the ways in which we interact than about the restrictions that constrain our actions. As in all things, there is a balance to achieve and unless we are in extremely constrained circumstances we have the means to generate some of the conditions in which creativity can flourish.

Ideas need mental space, not physical space. We can develop ideas by being aware of our surroundings and the dynamic nature of pressure to change. In health and social care services we can often recognise a need for change when we are aware of the experiences of service users. We can share ideas and build on them through conversation and listening. We can align our ideas with our shared values and gain wide commitment to making changes.

Dreams and visions of a better future arise from conditions in which creative ideas flourish. Some of the conditions that encourage creativity are:

- be open to the possibility of doing things differently;
- welcome challenge to the current ways of doing things – it forces consideration of change but does not, in itself, force change;
- avoid regulating any process that might have to be varied to be effective in different circumstances;
- encourage sharing of ideas;
- build on ideas rather than seeking to stifle them;
- be aware of and connect with your environment;
- be respectful of the ideas of others and seek to develop wider understanding;
- expect creativity and innovation to be a normal aspect of working together.

Openness to people and to your surroundings will often indicate opportunities to make helpful changes.

CREATIVE VISIONING

A vision is an idea that has been described in some way. It is not always a visual image, but might be described in words. One aspect of developing a vision is to turn an idea or a set of ideas into a coherent vision.

As an individual, you can use your own imagination and ability to be open to new ideas to develop your own vision. Shakti Gawain describes two ways in which we can do this for ourselves:

There are actually two different modes involved in creative visualization. One is the receptive, the other is active. In the receptive mode we simply relax and allow images or impressions to come to us without choosing the details of them; we take what comes. In the active mode we consciously choose and create what we wish to see or imagine. Both these processes are an important part of creative visualization, and your receptive and active abilities will both be strengthened through practice.

(Gawain, 1978, p. 27)

These two approaches provide a choice. People who are comfortable with working with their intuition and dreams can do so, and those who are more comfortable building on their ideas and making choices can take that approach. If we are working with groups, we will probably have to use both approaches if we are to welcome and respect all contributions.

Most approaches to visualisation that encourage you to be receptive require you to become very relaxed before allowing your mind to be open to ideas and impressions.

Example 10.1:   Relaxing

If the context permits, this can be done by lying on the floor, on your back, allowing your hands to turn upwards with the backs of your arms a little away from your body and your legs slightly apart.

You can then check each part of your body to deliberately relax the muscles. Do this by first taking your attention to your left foot. Tighten up the muscles in that foot, so that you can feel that they are tight. Then let all of the tightness go. Work your way to your ankle, your calf, your knee, your thigh, each time tightening the muscles and then letting the tightness go. Do this through the other leg, each arm; your abdomen, chest, back; your neck and face, until you have released the tension in all of your muscles and the floor is supporting your weight. Continue to breathe normally as you do this. Notice the rise and fall of your rib cage and the flow of air in and out of your lungs as you attempt to clear your mind.

You might need to practice this several times until you feel confident that you can bring yourself into a state of relaxation. This process, in itself, often enables people to open their minds by calming and soothing away the clamour of demands that so often surrounds us. You might stay in this relaxed position for a few minutes and try to keep your mind open to whatever might drift into it. If you find that day-to-day work keeps returning to you in a stressful way, you can maintain the relaxation by bringing your attention back to your body whenever you need to, returning to the checking process to let go of any tensions that have developed.

The relationship between relaxing and allowing vision to develop is not a direct one, because our busy lives sometimes keep intruding and demanding attention. There are some techniques that can help you to focus on developing your vision.

Some people find it helpful to use stories to set up the conditions in which they are open to receiving ideas. These often take the form of a short journey to a place where you will find a message. For example, you might imagine a walk through a wood to a clearing that becomes a special place for you and where you can be open to ideas. Other people might find it helpful to imagine a short boat journey to a special place. Use whatever imagery works for you and allow your story to have an 'open' space in it for you to discover something or to receive an idea. Then, again in your imagination, make your return journey and bring your attention back to your body and your surroundings. If you have had an idea or a message or a vision, make a note of it, even if you are not sure what it means. Sometimes it takes some time for complete ideas to develop and often they are more about our values or ways in which we do things in our lives than directly about different ways of organising our work.

We each have stories and symbols that are meaningful to us. One way of using this very directly is to visualise success when we are faced with something that we think is difficult. For example, if you have to make a formal presentation to a number of people and you are worried that your voice will dry up or your nerves will make you shake, visualise yourself performing the presentation smoothly and receiving warm applause. Do this as often as possible before the event.

Some people find that words and phrases work better for them than images. Spoken or written affirmations work strongly for some people. For example, if you frequently meet someone whose attitudes make you feel dismissed or overlooked, you might use a positive affirmation whenever you begin to feel overlooked. It might be worded something like, 'I make a valuable contribution through my work and my colleagues respect me.' You run this message through your mind whenever you begin to feel dismissed or whenever you need to remind yourself of the value of your work. Some people find that it is helpful to write messages of this type down and to put them in places where they will see them frequently.

One more technique that can be very helpful for people who hold onto anxieties and worries is to allow yourself to visualise them floating away. This is particularly helpful for worries that take your attention but that you cannot do anything about at the moment. The technique works by making a strong mental image of the anxiety, giving it a form as an image or as words. Then imagine putting it into a pink balloon that completely encases it. Allow the balloon to gently float away, bobbing up into the sky until it is out of sight. If you really must, you can keep hold of the end of a string so that you can pull the balloon back if you need to at some later date.

I warned you that creative visualisation is not something that appeals to everyone or that everyone will find possible or useful. There are other ways of developing vision and of incorporating ideas from others. It is important to remember, though, that we all bring different abilities and qualities to bear on our work and for most of us our work is an important part of our lives. If we respect what others offer, we are able to draw from a much broader resource than if we restrict development of ideas to a small group of people who think and develop ideas in similar ways.

SYSTEMS IN AN IDEAL WORLD

When we discussed rich pictures in Chapter 9 we left them at the point in which we had identified some focal areas that appeared to be opportunities to make improvements. This is not enough to provide a vision that will inspire action. We need to develop these ideas into something that describes a better future in a way that will be understood and supported by everyone involved. Look back at Figure 9.2. There are many people involved in different ways. There is also muddle in the range of demands and activities. The next stage in a systems thinking approach is to reduce the complexity so that we can view the situation as if it were in an ideal world.

First, consider what is supposed to be happening in the situation described in Figure 9.2. What is the primary task? Are there any secondary tasks? These are ones that support the primary task but are not part of it. The primary task is the prime purpose of the work in the setting described.

The purpose of the reception function in Figure 9.2 is to provide appointments for patients to meet with the two doctors and the nurse and to keep records relating to these appointments for each patient. This is the most important task, the reason why the reception function exists. In order to do this work the staff answer telephones, provide face-to-face information and a waiting area, file and retrieve individual patient records and arrange appointment times with the doctors and the nurse. There are other things happening that are secondary tasks, including the work of the Practice Manager in this context. It is important to remember the wider context when considering the primary task. In this case, the focus is on how patients receive the primary care service from the doctors or nurse.

In an ideal world, what would a system look like that enabled patients to meet their doctors or nurse when they wanted to consult with them? At this stage you can forget about the situation in the rich picture and simply think about what activities need to happen. If we start by thinking about the inputs, we have patients, staff (including the doctors, nurse and receptionists), information (including records), equipment (including telephones) and accommodation (including spaces for the staff, for patients to wait and for consultations to take place). What would we expect the outputs to be? We would expect each patient to have had a consultation and, ideally, for them to be satisfied with the outcome even if they did not find themselves completely returned to good health. We might want to define the outcomes more closely to set targets for minimum waiting times or for each patient to see their own doctor and we might also want to insist that the record keeping is accurate, up to date and available when needed.

Once we have identified the inputs and the outputs we can be specific about the transformation that has to take place to achieve the outputs. In this case, the patients need to have their request for an appointment received and processed to ensure that they are offered an appointment with the right doctor or the nurse within the specified minimum waiting time. The patient needs to arrive at the right time for their appointment and to have their consultation with the doctor or nurse. The doctor (or nurse) needs to have the patient records to provide information for each consultation. These records need to be updated as a result of the consultation and subsequently filed away for future reference. There may also be other tasks to carry out as a result of the consultation. For example, blood tests might have to be sent to a local laboratory. These are not necessarily tasks that have to be considered as part of the primary system if the outputs are only concerned with providing the opportunity for consultation. These additional tasks might be secondary to the primary tasks and associated with them or they might be part of separate but linked systems. In this case, we have not considered the work of other people in the practice or the other systems that will contribute to completing a much more complex set of outputs.

To continue with consideration of this single system, we might now describe the transformation system in its component steps:

1 Patient requests an appointment with their doctor.
2 Receptionist identifies an appropriate appointment time with the right doctor and agrees this with the patient.
3 Patient arrives for appointment as agreed.
4 Receptionist retrieves patient records and gives these to the doctor.
5 The consultation takes place, the doctor and patient agree a course of action and the records are updated.
6 The patient leaves.
7 The doctor returns the records to the receptionist to be filed away.

This sounds simple and straightforward, so why isn't life in the real world like this? The next stage in the process is to compare this ideal picture of the system with the rich picture and ask why the real world system does not operate as smoothly as it does in the ideal world. This usually needs to be considered in a discussion with those who are involved. The rich picture is only a starting point and will not have brought up all of the issues that need to be considered. Not everyone was involved in drawing this rich picture, so it would not necessarily be a good starting point for a discussion. The 'ideal' system can be used as a starting point by asking whether this does represent all of the steps that make up the system or whether there is anything that has been missed. Often people will suggest missing elements such as lack of time or resources, in which case it might be helpful to include discussion of the inputs and outputs to this system. Diagrams would probably be helpful for some people and the 'ideal' system can be drawn as a flow chart. In effect, this discussion is the opportunity to develop a vision of a better way of working.

This is also an opportunity to consider some possibilities that might improve things but that need discussion. It is helpful to avoid thinking that there is a technological solution for things, but when there is a need for accurate and shared record keeping, computers should be considered. For example, if the records were to be moved into an electronic system, they could be retrieved by each doctor or by the nurse when the patient was with them. They could also be updated and refiled immediately. The 'cost' of this would be that a system would have to be provided and everyone would have to learn how to use it. In many primary care settings this has been achieved in a way that provides advantages in managing other information requirements. Sometimes it is difficult to consider making significant change in one system without also noting the implications for others.

This approach can offer a practical and systematic way of developing a vision. Use of diagrams and charts can help groups of people to share understanding and to work towards solutions to the problems that they discuss. Keeping an emphasis on the outputs can be helpful in focusing on improvement. If the people involved in the setting have been part of discussing the existing situation and the possibilities, they will be likely to want to support change.

RECONCILING ALTERNATIVE VISIONS

As change in one area often has implications for other areas of work, there may be different ideas about what a better situation would look like. People in one area of work might have focused their thinking on how to improve the physical conditions in which they work. Others might have focused on making improvements to the ways in which they work, and people in another area might have put more emphasis on the interactions and communications that take place within their area of work. This can be a great advantage, because these ideas can be brought together to create a much richer vision that can attract the support of many more people.

If no attempt is made to bring different visions together, there is a danger that momentum to change will be lost while people compete to support different visions. When one group of people have developed a vision they can become quite possessive about it. Involvement at this stage of any other people who will be affected by the proposed change can enable a more inclusive vision to be developed. This will also ensure that more people are ready to support the changes.

COMMITTING TO THE VISION

The process of developing the vision is not complete until enough people become committed to the vision to provide support for change. The process of developing commitment has been described as circling frequently and closing as late as possible. The circling has probably already taken place in the form of discussion and development of ideas with different individuals and groups and then with larger groups, perhaps from different areas of work. To ensure that everyone stays in touch with the vision as it becomes more detailed and more widely understood, the original groups need to continue to be involved. It is helpful to stay open to minor alterations and embellishments to the vision for as long as possible.

Communication during development of the vision is very important. Even if there is wide involvement in developing a shared vision, those who have not been part of the latest discussion will want to be kept informed and consulted about any proposed additions or alterations. Those who have been involved in discussions will probably talk to others, so an informal sharing of information will shape understanding alongside whatever formal communications are shared. Sometimes use of flip charts as ideas sheets in convenient places in organisations can allow ideas to be offered for consideration at later meetings. News-sheets outlining progress and inviting other ideas can help to both keep the lines of communication open and involve those who cannot take part in the group discussions. Two-way communications are essential if those developing the vision are to stay aware of any discomfort or dissent. Challenges to the developing vision are often very useful in pointing out weaknesses or ideas that are unlikely to gain wider support. Effective communications during the development of vision will both share ideas and enable ideas to be questioned and challenged.

When the vision seems to be fairly complete and robust in describing a desirable future that is widely supported, the process of developing the vision will have made strong connections between the past, the present and the imagined future. You will be able to describe this connection as a story that can help to prepare everyone for the change process. The story will have a beginning. This may include acknowledgement of past success and strengths in the organisation and lead to how people began to realise that change was necessary. The story might then continue to note the key issues that were discussed and the opinions that were expressed during consultations about possible futures. The story might describe the contradictions that emerged and the difficulties that were faced in attempting to reconcile different views. A compelling story will weave these elements to arrive at a description of the future that everyone agrees will be the right next step. This story will be the one that is repeated throughout the change process to inform and to inspire progression towards its conclusion.

Development of a vision is more than setting a goal that sets a marker for change. It can be a process that engages people's hopes and fears, that involves people in revisiting their values and facing challenges to their assumptions. The reward for engaging in a process that involves people in this way is the commitment that is generated. This commitment can provide the energy and willingness to try different ways of working that are essential to carry out change.

CHAPTER 11

DEVELOPING DIRECTION

This chapter brings us to strategy and planning. The focus is on what needs to be done to develop a direction that will enable the transformation to take place to achieve your vision. As we have seen in previous chapters, the transformation is unlikely to be something that can be achieved with a single straight pathway. Changing the ways we do things involves revisiting our values and those of our organisation. We need to consider how to progress in a way that will align the various elements to create the new conditions.

The vision is usually redefined as a set of key objectives, in order to begin strategic planning. The strategy provides a framework for planning the details. It also allows the overall ideas to be shared in a way that fits into the normal work of your organisation. Planning is also a normal activity and there are numerous techniques that can help you to develop your plans. Plans, however, are temporary and need to be frequently revised and updated. In complex change we sometimes need to consider having several sets of plans for alternative possibilities.

In planning change it is very important to consider people; how much to involve them and when, how they might feel about proposals and how to communicate the plans so that everyone understands what is proposed and why. There is almost always some resistance to change and this will usually be evident during the planning stage and during the change processes. There are various ways in which we can work with resistance and some advantages in encouraging dissident voices during the planning stage. This will allow different views to be considered and perhaps to shape the planning. Ideally, planning and communication about change will also include development of support for the plans.

Once the direction has been developed, there is a further communication requirement, as everyone will need to know what they have to do in order to make progress. Knowing what is required and doing it are, of course, different things. We conclude this chapter by reviewing what is needed to equip people to take action and consider what inspires people to do these things in the following chapter.

PREPARING FOR TRANSITION

Transformation involves a period of transition while the change is taking place. In health and care services we are rarely able to suspend service provision while we make a change, so we usually need to plan to continue provision and to make the transition to the new conditions alongside each other. This does not necessarily mean that everything continues to be done in the same way until the magic moment when the change can happen, at which stage everything changes. Usually we make the transition in stages or even in parallel processes where change happens at different times in each of the different systems that comprise the transforming service.

There are choices to make about what is to be done and how it is to be done. The vision will probably give an incomplete idea of what is to be achieved, so there will be many details to consider. One of the key choices to make in developing direction is the choice of who should be involved. It may be practical to have a small team developing the strategy and plans, but the members of this team might be selected for their skills or for their ability to represent different views in the organisation. You might choose to do both of these in a core team but also to consult widely. If you do consult widely, you need to consider the extent to which the results of consultation will be allowed to shape the planning process. If people are consulted and see that their input has not been acknowledged, they will soon lose confidence in what will appear to be only a pretence of involvement.

Developing direction is essentially about clarifying the purpose of change and agreeing how we'll make the transition. In a complex environment it is not about identifying one clear pathway but about identifying a number of pathways that twist and turn around the obstacles. Clarity of purpose is important, as this will provide some broad guidance about both the way in which we travel and how to progress in the right direction. The values that underpin the vision of how we want to change are also crucial in providing a framework that will enable decisions to be made.

ALIGNING VALUES

Change stimulates us to revisit some of the important values that underpin our work and to consider to what extent our personal values are aligned with these. We sometime assume that our values are at one with the prevalent organisational values. In practice, there are often differences that have not been recognised or understood. Sometimes the gap between our own values and the values that underpin our work has widened without our having recognised the gradual change. When we develop a vision as preparation for a change in an organisation, we incorporate values in the vision. The vision is the picture of what we want to achieve. Vision and values are closely connected because a vision of a better future is inevitably coloured by values that view one state as more desirable than another. We may have discussed these values whilst developing the vision. We may have made adaptations to accommodate differences of opinion without attempting to reconcile different values. As we move closer to change in developing strategy and plans, we will have to reconsider the values that underpin the vision of the future and reconcile these with the values that are inherent in our current work. If these do not easily align, we may have to consider which are the right values to underpin our future work.

Values are deep-seated beliefs about what is right or wrong and what is important and unimportant. An organisation's values are influenced both by values held in the wider world within which it functions and also by values held by all the people who work in it and who use its services. In thinking about values, it is helpful to consider these different levels.

The values of a society influence organisations and an organisation's values influence the values of teams and individuals within it. But the influence also passes upwards; individuals influence their groups, their organisations and the society in which they live.

A useful mnemonic is SOGI, representing the values of:

- Society;
- Organisation;
- Group or team;
- Individual.

INFLUENCE OF VALUES

Values vary enormously in different countries, communities and cultures. Modern industrial societies include communities with very different values, living and working together in ways regulated by society as a whole. Frequently there are tensions between different values in a mixed community. In the United Kingdom, for example, there is a tension between the extent to which a 'free market' is allowed to shape the ways in which people live and work and the extent to which public services are funded by taxpayers to provide essential services.

Public services are very much influenced by the values of the government in power. Public services have been criticised for being bureaucratic, over-centralised and dominated by professionals. There has also been increasing pressure for more attention to be paid to the views of users of public services. A number of pressure groups, with their own demands, emerged during the 1980s. This trend was supported by many professionals, particularly those working in social care who wanted to work in different ways and who were often unhappy about the inflexibility and unaccountability that charac-terised many of the organisations in which they worked. New kinds of support services emerged that demonstrated different ways of working. For example, women's organisations set up support groups in the form of rape crisis centres, and gay and lesbian organisations set up telephone helplines. These established different relation-ships between service users and service providers, met needs that had previously been ignored, and were often run in more collaborative ways than traditional services. As Sang commented:

> The proliferation of groups, networks and formally constituted organisations is astonishing. One London primary care group identified more than 300 service user and carer groups in its locality, and the College of Health has more than 2,500 self-help and service user groups on its database ... There is a real opportunity to be seized – and a real threat to be challenged. For if this movement is not recognised and appropriately valued, then patients, clients and carers will see only tokenism and betrayal – not the 'partnership' that is so often, so rhetorically and so frequently proclaimed.
>
> (Sang, 1999, pp. 22–23)

Tensions between professionals, service users and the public were exacerbated by concerns that people who were entrusted with responsibility for public funds were not always putting the interests of the public before their personal interests. Lord Nolan was asked to convene a committee to consider and report on the expectations that the public might reasonably have of those holding responsible positions in government or public services.

Example 11.1:   Values underpinning public service

The Nolan Committee was particularly concerned with setting principles for those who hold senior and influential positions in public life, but the values expressed in these principles might be considered appropriate for anyone with any level of responsibility in public service:

- Selflessness – People in public service should act solely in the public interest. They should not gain financial or other material benefits for themselves, their family or their friends.
- Integrity – People in public service should not place themselves under any financial or other obligation to outside individuals or organisations that might seek to influence them in the performance of their official duties.
- Objectivity – People in public service should make choices on merit in carrying out public business, including making public appointments, awarding contracts or recommending individuals for rewards and benefits.
- Accountability – People in public service are accountable to the public for their decisions and actions and must submit themselves to whatever scrutiny is appropriate to their role.
- Openness – People in public service should be as open as possible about all the decisions and actions that they take. They should give reasons for their decisions and restrict information only when the wider public interest clearly demands it.
- Honesty – People in public service have a duty to declare any private interests relating to their public duties and to take steps to resolve any conflicts that may arise in a way that protects the public interest.

■ Leadership – People in public service should promote and support these principles by leadership and example.
(adapted from the report of the Nolan Committee, 1996)

This statement of principles is helpful in making the notion of a 'public service ethic' more explicit.

You might have been in a situation in which you have been concerned about one of these principles in relation to your own values and role. You might have been offered a free lunch by someone who hoped to be rewarded by your support for a decision to purchase their drugs or equipment. You might have been asked to help someone to jump the queue for a service or you may have been offered a reward if you would give someone preferential treatment. It is more difficult to be selfless in a situation like this if you see a member of your own family having to queue when in pain and waiting for an operation.

If you are working in health or care in the voluntary or private sector, your service users may also expect you and your organisation to demonstrate values similar to those expressed by the Nolan Committee's principles. They will also expect selflessness, integrity, objectivity, accountability, openness, honesty and leadership to be evident. Within society as a whole, people who work in various professions and occupations also often have their own sets of values which, though drawing on broader societal values, have their own particular characteristics. These are often expressed in the form of codes of ethics or statements of values or standards. The multi-occupational and multi-agency nature of health and social care means that different sets of values can be seen within a single organisation or between organisations that are working collaboratively to deliver a coherent service to patients or service users. Sometimes there are conflicts between the priorities expressed in the values of different groups. For example, keeping to appointment times in clinics may be seen by doctors as less important than taking enough time to give full attention to the patient in front of them. The focus on the individual patient may sometimes lead to a tension between delivery of a service to one person and delivery of that service to many people.

Organisations in the health and social care sector are guided by values expressed at a national level as government policies. Usually there is an emphasis on standards and accountability, both of which are concerns in the public, private and voluntary sectors. Values may be specific in mentioning both standards in relation to the results achieved by services and standards of care and respect for people, as well as improving standards through research and education. Value statements may mention achievement of national standards being a local responsibility and high-quality care that delivers excellence to all patients. Often there is indication of a concern to meet local needs while contributing to wider health improvements. Values may be explicit about responsiveness, requiring services to identify and seek to meet people's needs and wishes, which indicates a concern to listen to a wider public voice than that of patients and service users. Health and care organisations might also state an aim to enable staff to work purposefully while feeling valued and sharing the values of the service.

All of these themes are related to modernising services to work in ways that fit more closely with public expectations as well as meeting national and local needs. The themes that emerge are relevant to all areas of public services and are central to the aim of providing integrated services rather than separate specialist services. People who are working in health services, for example, can expect to work more closely in future with people in social care, housing and education. There is an increasing emphasis on making sure that services are 'joined up' and do not leave patients and service users with their needs only partially met.

The Institute for Public Policy Research (1999) identified eight values that provide a national health service with its 'moral base':

- Good health – a commitment to improving the nation's health;
- Efficiency in the use of public resources – treatments should provide high value relative to opportunity costs;
- Equity – with recognition that this is a major issue given the climate of priority-setting and rationing;
- Choice – the state should allow some degree of personal choice for individuals;
- Democracy – the service should be publicly accountable for the quality of service provision;
- Respect for human dignity – the relationship between the provider and the receiver of health care should reflect this;
- Public service – includes some of the above but also covers 'altruism rather than profit' and the notion that health service staff should work for the common good;
- Universality – a service for all, paid for by everyone via taxation, is essential to provide security and reassurance to the population and to foster social cohesion.

The Institute's report acknowledged that some of these values conflict with one other: for example, patient choice versus efficiency. The public may place a much higher value on access to a local hospital threatened with closure than on higher-quality outcomes for a small group of patients with a particular condition.

This list of values relates to a national health service as a whole, but you will probably also be able to identify organisational values in relation to the unit or department in which you work. However, within a large organisation such as a hospital or a social services department, the extent to which staff are aware of and influenced by organisational values can vary enormously. A junior doctor or social worker may be completely unaware of the hospital's or department's values and may identify far more readily with the values of his or her medical college or professional association. In addition, sometimes there is inconsistency between the values that an organisation tries to uphold and those that it demonstrates in its actions. This is sometimes referred to as the difference between an organisation's *espoused* values and its *enacted* values.

Within health and social care organisations, there is usually a complex array of staff teams comprising people from many occupational areas. Teams that work together regularly often adopt common values that focus on the purpose of their work and recognise the contribution made by team members who bring particular and different skills. As public services are encouraged to develop more integrated provision and to work more closely together, the values underlying principles and mission statements need to be more widely discussed and considered from a number of perspectives if they are to be implemented across services.

Those who work in multi-agency or multi-professional teams often have to deal with situations in which there are conflicting or competing values. In such situations it may be necessary to reinterpret core values in the new setting. This might be achieved by establishing agreement over a more inclusive set of values, for example by focusing on what the service is aiming to deliver or on broader public service values.

Our personal values are also significant in our approach to working with others. Our values arise from the values of our social background, our religion (if we have one), our ethnic origin or subculture, our upbringing and education, and our experience of life and work. They continue to develop and change throughout our lives as we encounter new and contradictory situations and reflect on our experiences. Our early values are based on the culture in which we grew up, often in the narrow confines of a family or social group. It is not until we experience unfamiliar settings that we encounter views and behaviours that surprise us or, sometimes, offend us. We then have opportunities to consider the values that we hold which cause us to respond as we do. These are often the moments that lead to transformative learning, after which we become more aware of the beliefs that inform our viewpoints. Some people are very aware of their values and how they use them when making judgements, but others make judgements without questioning the value base that underpins them. We are all individuals and we are all different. No wonder that it is sometimes difficult for an individual to fit in with a group or an organisation!

Individual values fit broadly into two types:

- values about how you think things should be done;
- values about goals.

Values about how things should be done include working hard and being honest, open-minded, fair, forgiving, respectful of differences, supportive of equality. Values about goals include happiness, prosperity, well-being, accomplishments and self-respect. The personal challenge is to understand your own values and why you hold them so that you can be more aware of how other people are driven by their values. If you can recognise the differences and tensions that arise from value conflicts, you are more likely to be able to help to resolve them.

The challenge for change agents is to be aware of the values that underpin the views that people express. Change is essentially about both how things are done and the goals that are implicit in the vision of the future. It is often possible to secure agreement over the core values of service delivery and to work from that agreement to an understanding of how individuals and teams can contribute to the work of the organisation without feeling that their values are being compromised. If you challenge another person's values, you may appear to be challenging very personal issues and may seem to be undermining another person's identity.

If we are to be successful in leading change, we need to work within the values of our organisation. We also need to be aware of our own values, the values held by the various individuals and teams in our areas of work and those held by patients, service users and carers.

DEVELOPING A PLAN FOR CHANGE

Change in any part of an organisation is only likely to gain wide support if it makes a contribution to achieving the overall purpose and goals of the organisation. It also needs to do so in a way that embodies the values of the organisation. Before making a plan for change in any part of your service, you need to review the most recent documents in your organisation that detail the overall strategy and the policies that guide the ways in which things are done. With these in mind, you can redefine the vision to describe it as a service or part of a service, including a statement about how it contributes to achieving the aims of the organisation.

Strategy is about redefining the vision as a set of aims and then identifying the ways in which progress will be made towards achieving these aims. There are, therefore, two important aspects to a strategic framework for planning: the statements that describe the aims and objectives and statements that describe how these will be achieved. Sometimes the vision can be translated into aims that are already well defined and can probably be achieved fairly quickly. In this case a plan for change can follow logical steps.

There is a sequence of questions that you need to answer to produce the steps in an outline plan for change:

1 What are we trying to achieve?
2 What is the best way of doing it?
3 What tasks and activities are involved?
4 In what order should we do these?
5 What resources do we need?
6 How shall we review progress?
7 Who will do what and when?

These questions should help you to plan how to move from where you are through the changes that will bring you to the new state represented in the vision. Let us consider each of these questions and the way in which you might develop answers.

Step 1. What are we trying to achieve?

The answer to this question should be the aims and key objectives that, when you put them together, add up to achieving the new state described in the vision. You might already have identified these aims and objectives as part of the process of defining the vision. It is important to include every aspect of the vision that contributes to it being distinctly different from the current conditions. For example, if one aspect of the vision is to deliver services to patients in a way that avoids long queues or waiting lists, you need to state this and have a clear idea of how that will be achieved. If it is an aspiration but there are no ideas about how it might be delivered, you can either spend more time in generating ideas and discussing possibilities or amend the vision to something that is achievable, perhaps appointment systems within a target time.

There is no point in starting to develop plans if the vision does not seem possible to achieve. It is more practical to allow the aspiration, the dream, to sit as a future hope and to use it to help to develop direction towards it. This will mean that you have to bring a practical element into discussions now and work towards agreement about what can be achieved within a reasonable time. It is not usually helpful to extend the time for change to allow more to be achieved – it is more satisfying for everyone to aim for something that is achievable within a few months. An achievement will usually set the tone for further development and give everyone confidence to engage in further change. There is also an advantage in not setting too long a time-scale because the environmental conditions that affect your organisation and service area will change over time and you will want to keep any internal changes flexible to respond to the new requirements.

If you realise that it will not be possible to achieve the vision in one step change, be careful to discuss this fully with everyone involved. If the vision has attracted support and enthusiasm for action, people will be disappointed if it seems that too little is to be attempted. They would also be disappointed, however, if too much is attempted and nothing achieved. This first question needs to be thought about carefully and agreement reached about how big a step might be taken. If there is to be more than one step, it is helpful to keep the further steps visible in any planning discussions so that thinking is focused on steps towards a future that is attractive and worthwhile.

Step 2. What is the best way of doing it?

This is a big question because it includes defining the processes that you will use, considering whether these adequately demonstrate your values and how you will communicate. You will remember that people may hold strong values about the ways in which we do things. You may not be aware of the implications of these values until you propose a course of action and discover that, for a number of different reasons, people raise objections. Situations in which proposals are challenged or rejected can be largely avoided if enough consultation is carried out before firm proposals are made. Consultation needs to include anyone who will be affected by the change as well as those whose co-operation will be necessary to carry out the change.

'Making the right sort of space for development – physical, social and psychological – is an essential task for all organizational "architects" who are interested in creating the Learning Company. Noisy manufacturing processes, over-controlled hierarchies and crowded premises can all block the opportunities for risk and reflection needed for learning.' (Pedler, Burgoyne and Boydell, 1991, p. 67)

You might distinguish between these groups. If development of the vision has raised enthusiasm and there are people wanting to make progress, these might be the ones who could lead consultation about how to progress by first gaining support for the ideas and then asking for suggestions about the ways in which progress might be achieved. It is much easier to progress consultation in this way when a proposal for change has support at all levels and people willing to shape opinion. Often it is difficult for senior people to ask for suggestions about how to achieve a vision, especially in an organisation where there is tight control and regulation. Change agents can operate in highly regulated conditions but they need the support of senior people so that they can champion the cause without becoming martyrs for it. Change almost always involves challenging the existing conditions and in highly regulated organisations this is not welcome behaviour. We should note that it is not welcome behaviour in most organisations and change agents always need support unless they are ready to risk a great deal.

Another aspect of finding out more at this stage is to check whether there is any evidence that supports choice of a particular way of doing things. You might check whether anyone has done anything like this before. Reports of change within your own organisation can be very helpful, particularly if the lessons that were learnt are noted. Reports from similar organisations can also be helpful if you allow for the differences in conditions. You might also check whether there is a best practice model, as people who have been successful in carrying out a change similar to the one you propose will often be willing to discuss their experience with you. You could also enquire whether there is any benchmark information relevant to your proposed change that might help you to set objectives and standards that others have found achievable. Any evidence you can obtain that supports either the proposed aims or the choice of processes to achieve the aims will be helpful in gaining wide support for investment in change.

When change is proposed in complex service settings a number of options often emerge, particularly when consultation has been extensive. It is often tempting to dismiss some options that, in your own opinion, are unsuitable or unlikely to succeed. If you do this, you might find that it is hard to progress the change because people involved feel that decisions were made too quickly or without due consideration. It is usually helpful to generate a number of options and then to be very open about how a decision is made. A 'transparent' way of making a decision is to set criteria for the judgement. These should reflect the values and the aims that are embodied in the vision. A process can then be developed to enable the choice to be made. Appropriate processes are described in more detail in Martin (2002, pp. 27–36).

The ways in which we do things shape what can be done. The processes chosen to progress ideas influence the outcomes. It is very important to ensure that you choose ways of working that enable change. If you attempt to make change by using existing structures and ways of working, you will often find that the processes replicate the present state and do not allow change into the future state that you are attempting to achieve. This is why there has been so much emphasis on restructuring and on designing processes that do what we want them to do (process re-engineering). If you think about the idea of an ideal system (discussed in Chapter 9) you can check that the processes you choose for change represent a clear sequence of steps to transform the inputs into the outputs that are needed to achieve your aims.

I have mentioned the possibility that the change might not be achieved. Once the overall plan is agreed, there will be enough information available to carry out a risk assessment. This requires a different type of thinking from the creative thinking that has been part of developing the vision and attracting support. As soon as you begin to think about investing time and money in the initiative, there are risks to be considered. Your organisation may be able to provide help in carrying out a risk assessment. If you need to set something up for yourself, there is further information about managing risk and impact assessment in Martin (2002, pp. 52–61).

Step 3. What tasks and activities are involved?

Once the broad decisions are made about process, this stage can be one that involves everyone who will be contributing to making the change. If the people who are to do the work plan how they will do it, they will have ownership of the process and be much more likely to do it with enthusiasm.

If the change will involve several teams it is helpful to divide the work into objectives and to identify the main activities that will have to be completed to achieve the objectives. Once teams have been established to take responsibility for each of these activity areas, the work can be subdivided into tasks. Agreement can then be gained about who will carry out each task and estimates can be made about how long the task will take.

Step 4. In what order should we do these?

As you begin to talk about individual tasks that contribute to achieving objectives, it becomes clear that some things cannot be started until others are complete. We usually need to schedule tasks in each activity area to ensure that we make good use of people's time and energy. Once there is a schedule of tasks and activities, we have a time line that indicates how long the whole change will take. This can be surprising and sometimes raises questions about how the change could be accomplished more quickly. It often takes much longer than had been anticipated to carry out the work that will be the foundation for further work. It is only when detailed estimates are prepared that the whole sequence of necessary tasks can be seen.

There are some ways in which the processes can be speeded up. For example, we could put more people to work on the initial tasks. Or we could increase the time that is spent on the initial tasks by extending the working day. We might decide that a lower quality of work or outcomes would be acceptable and achievable in a shorter time. Our options are usually to invest more time or money or to change the quality requirements. These concerns are faced by anyone managing projects in health or social care and are discussed more fully in Martin (2002).

Step 5. What resources do we need?

The scheduling of activities and tasks can be used to identify the resource needs for each activity. If you need to maintain a service while change is taking place, this will also need to be considered. Be careful not to overload staff by expecting them to work on the new activities at the same time as they continue with their existing work. Although most people are willing to make a special effort for a short time, asking people to carry an overload for any length of time brings risks to the individuals and to the change initiative if people become ill and unable to work. It would also be an expectation that many would find did not embody the values that they had supported in the proposed change.

Therefore we should expect there to be a cost. If the change is worthwhile, the cost will lead to benefits that justify the use of resources. If we are convinced of the value of change, we should not be shy about requesting resources. If the change is significant, people from the personnel and finance departments will probably need to be involved.

Step 6. How shall we review progress?

The most important issue in planning a way to review progress is to establish how you will know what is happening. You might simply ask teams to report progress in completion of tasks and processes. You could then compare this with the schedule to ensure that every-thing progresses as planned. This is unlikely in a complex setting when other activities may impact on the planned change, so some provision has to be made to revise the plans when necessary. A more formal process of setting targets for key outcomes to be achieved by specific dates might be necessary to enable you to manage resources, particularly when one set of activities depends on another set being completed at a particular time. These techniques are also those needed in project management.

Another question that is important in a change initiative is how you will know that the progress that is being made is achieving what was intended. This is a more general question than those asked about specific targets because it concerns the overall outcome of the activity. You might identify indicators of success that can be used to discuss progress. The most important thing is to ensure that all the effort and resource is focused on achieving the future that you intend to achieve and not something that emerges as a result of poorly focused activity.

You might also consider when to review and who should be involved. There is often a need for some formal and some informal opportunities to discuss progress. There might be specific achieve-ments at some stages of the work that can be celebrated as success. This can be helpful in reviving confidence and commitment.

Step 7. Who will do what and when?

The decisions about who will do what and when are mostly taken when the activities and tasks are allocated and scheduled, but there are some additional management tasks in planning and managing the processes, including reviews and revision of plans. There will also probably be some formal procedures to enable work to start and to deal with resources.

PLANNING IN LESS CERTAIN CONDITIONS

The seven planning steps work well when the change we are planning has clear goals so that aims and objectives can be set. When the goals are not so clear, or the conditions in which we are working are subject to sudden change, it is less realistic to plan a continuous sequence of activities. Our planning takes place in a tension between what we believe is certain and what is uncertain. It is also subject to what we believe we can control and what we cannot control. These dimensions can be used to set up a matrix that outlines four positions in which we might find ourselves (Figure 11.1).

As you see in Figure 11.1, there are four boxes with different characteristics determined by the vertical and horizantal dimensions. Box 1 represents a position in which the conditions are certain, well known and understood. We know what needs to change and we have the control to make changes. In this position you can use planning methods that assume fairly constant conditions. Change can be managed as a normal part of working life. Project management methods will work well in this situation. Although plans always need some revison and change, the conditions in which the change is happening are unlikely to change enough to cause a need for drastic revision or to threaten the initiative. This all sounds rather secure

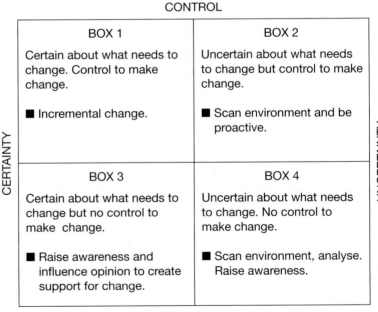

Figure 11.1   Approaches to planning change

and comforting, so it is worth mentioning that the main danger in this position is that we might think we are there because we have not noticed the uncertainties or because we think we have control that in reality we do not have.

Box 2 also represents a position in which we have significant control, but in this box we are aware that there are uncertainties in our environment. We can, however, identify many of these uncertainties as the forces driving change: social, technical, economic, environmental and political pressures. As we have control we can identify the pressures that are most likely to impact on our area of work and prepare our organisation to change in response to the pressure. In this way we can be proactive in deciding how we will respond and we can reshape our services in a way that we want them to develop.

In Box 3 we have no control over making changes but we are certain about conditions that are putting pressure on our organisation or area of work and what needs to change. This is a position in which we can visualise what we might do but we find ourselves unable to make changes to achieve the vision. In this position we have no control but we can raise awareness of the pressures to change. We can use influence and persuasion to try to encourage people to make changes that will respond to the pressures. We can work with the informal power within our organisation or area of work to try to change attitudes and to develop an attractive vision of change that people will be willing to work towards. You will not be able to use change or project management techniques that require formal controls, but you might be able to use these techniques with the consent of colleagues if they can see the benefits of organising work collectively to achieve changes that they all accept are desirable.

In Box 4 we are in the position of being uncertain about what needs to change and unable to make changes. We can choose not to be in this position. Anyone can make an analysis of the environmental situation (see Chapter 8) and can try to raise awareness within their organisation or area of work. If nothing is done to make changes, the pressures to change will cause reactive response or complete inability to function. This can lead to an organisation being seen to fail to achieve its prime purpose or it might be closed down if it becomes unfit to work at all. For example, an organisation may be so slow to react that essential targets have not been met. Or new legislation might require adaptations to buildings to be made by a certain date after which any organisation that is unable to comply will be unable to continue to work.

This matrix can be used to help us to identify the position our organisation or service is in, in relation to awareness of the need to change and control over making changes. The way in which we approach planning change will be different in each of these circumstances. In Box 1 the degree of awareness and control can provide considerable support for change, for change agents and for those leading change. In Box 2 more emphasis needs to be placed on developing an understanding of the pressures to change so that decisions can be made to make changes. The control systems are there to support planning and implementation of change once the decisions are made. In Box 3 the problem is one of how to initiate and control change in a situation where people are not used to having their work controlled. This can often be overcome by raising awareness and facilitating discussion until enough agreement has been reached to progress change through negotiation and individual effort.

If you are in Box 4, your organisation or area of work is threatened by its lack of awareness and inability to control change. Although you can identify the main drivers of change and explain how these are likely to impact on the organisation, this might not be enough to raise awareness. Scenario planning offers a method of considering the future that is often helpful in complex settings where the impacts of environmental pressure are not easy to understand.

A SWOT analysis of your organisation in relation to its current environment will consider:

■ Strengths
■ Weaknesses
■ Opportunities
■ Threats

in terms of how the weaknesses might be strengthened and the threats reduced by taking some of the opportunities.

Scenarios are essentially stories about the future. You can create scenarios by taking one of the pressures for change and developing the story about what will happen as it becomes stronger. Perhaps imagine the scenario as it might be one year ahead and then in three years' time. For each of these periods, outline the environmental conditions as they will have changed as the force for change gathers momentum and check how your organisation might perform in those conditions. You can use the SWOT approach by asking what opportunities and threats have emerged in the new conditions and then ask what your organisation's strengths and weaknesses are in relation to these scenarios. The implications might be brought into sharp focus by asking key individuals in your organisation to take part in a scenario discussion in which they are each asked what they would do if they found themselves in the new conditions. It soon becomes apparent whether there is a need for change or not.

COMMUNICATING THE DIRECTION

If you have developed the direction with wide involvement, many people will already be aware of the intention to change and may know something about the plans. There will be other people who need to be informed and possibly more consultation to carry out once the plans have been developed in some detail. Change will be much easier to accomplish if people are broadly in agreement with the goals of the change and the way in which it is to be carried out.

A plan can be used to facilitate communication. It can help the organisation to explain its intentions to patients, service users and other customers. The plan can also help us to communicate our future intentions to other organisations with which we have contacts of various types. It can also help us to communicate to the general public what the organisation is planning to do in order to improve the services offered.

The plans will also be needed to prepare for implementation of change. Everyone who will be involved needs to know what they are expected to do and when this needs to be done. People need both to know what is expected and to be willing to start work. Sometimes more has to be done to create the conditions in which people are both ready to start and equipped adequately to take on their individual tasks.

This chapter has focused on developing direction. We have considered how values underpin our attitudes towards both the goals that are set and the processes that are used in making changes. We have taken an overview of a planning process that can be used when aims and objectives can be set. We have also considered situations in which planning is not so easily accomplished. We concluded by mentioning the importance of communicating plans to those who will be affected by the change and those who will be involved in making the change. The next chapter looks at how we can inspire and facilitate people to take action.

CHAPTER 12

INSPIRING ACTION

The process of developing direction leads to a plan for action, but it is usually necessary to revive enthusiasm for the vision in order to inspire people to take action. In this chapter we focus on both how to initiate progress towards achieving our aims and how to keep up the momentum once we have started.

There are two aspects to this implementation stage: keeping up morale and enthusiasm, and managing the process in relation to the plan. We focus on the leadership aspects of this stage more than on the management issues, but these are noted because they provide essential reassurance and information.

Most of the issues that arise in leading change are the result of differences in expectations. Even if we are sure that the processes in development of vision and direction explored the different views that people hold, the strength of these views often becomes much more apparent during implementation of change. One of the most important influences on people is organisational culture. We consider ways in which culture can influence change and what leaders and change agents can do to work with the issues.

We conclude the chapter by looking more carefully at resistance to change and considering what might be done to reduce the impact of resistance.

INSPIRING OTHERS

Once we arrive at the time when people can begin to make the changes that have been agreed, the focus moves to practicalities and the vision can seem dim and distant. We often need to remind ourselves why we have set out on this course and what we expect to gain as a result of the disruption that change inevitably brings.

Inspiration is an interesting word for the feeling that we have when we are enthusiastic and empowered. The word 'inspiration' really means taking in a breath, filling our lungs with life-giving air. In some cultures the act of breathing is recognised as a positive contribution to life and different ways of breathing are practiced as contributing to meditation. In Western civilisations breathing is usually considered to be one of the automatic behaviours and not something that we use in a deliberate way. We do, however, talk about taking a deep breath before doing something difficult. Inspiration provides strength.

You might have derived personal strength from your own passion if you care deeply about achieving the change. When we feel passionately about something we often try not to show it, particularly at work where it might feel rather silly to show that you care. We learn at an early age not to show our feelings when we are vulnerable, and most of us do feel vulnerable at work, especially when our emotions are strong and difficult to manage. In health and social care services staff often face tragic situations and are expected not to show their own feelings very strongly but to cope with the situation and to move on to work with the next set of events. It might not come easily to you to allow others to see your passion and commitment. It can, however, be very inspiring to others if you do allow your own feelings to show. You don't have to be a charismatic leader who can persuade by force of personality. People will find you inspiring if you can talk about a vision of a better future with energy and enthusiasm, showing in your eyes and voice that this is the future that you would like to work towards. You can support this by giving clear descriptions of what will be different and why it matters. Your personal commitment and clear reasoning will attract support.

You will keep that support if you prove to be trustworthy and a person of integrity. As people embark on a course of change they take a risk because they move away from familiar and safe ground. Be careful what promises and reassurance you offer because people will expect you to keep your promises. Promise only what you can, personally, deliver. Your integrity is demonstrated in the way that you behave. The ways in which you interact with other people, the respect that you show, your conscientiousness and your compassion all offer evidence of your integrity. The guidelines developed by the Nolan Committee (Example 11.1) provide some food for thought about personal integrity.

LEADING AND MANAGING THE PROCESS

During implementation of change, both your leadership and management skills are needed. Leadership is needed to inspire and challenge. Management is needed to provide resources, develop plans, monitor progress and manage the processes. These roles and responsibilities can be shared and do not need to be together in one person, but both roles are needed to effect change. Leaders will be needed to keep up morale and enthusiasm for change and managers will be needed to support planned progress and to collect and provide information about the extent to which targets are being met.

At an early stage in implementation you will need to ensure that you are empowered to act. You need to have support to initiate action and any resources that are necessary. Others who are to take action will also need support and resources. Some will need to be reassured about the extent to which they can make decisions and take action without supervision, particularly if they are used to working in a highly regulated situation. Those who demonstrate leadership in progressing change can be encouraged and supported to develop their abilities. Leaders learn to lead by doing it and reflecting on the results of their actions.

For everyone involved in change, there is an element of transition from the current state into the new state. Some will find this a more difficult experience than others. Some may find it hard to cope at times and some will need support if they feel incompetent when they begin to work in different ways. Some people will need training and development to be able to work in different ways and this should be provided when it is needed or in preparation for new roles. There will also be changes in the ways that people think about work if processes are changing. Opportunities may be needed to test out ideas and to review new ideas in groups and teams. There may also be opportunities to share learning and know-how as some people begin to develop new ways of doing things. Emotions will often be easily roused during change and everyone might be encouraged to try to treat each other with respect and to respect dignity (particularly in situations where people might feel foolish if they are not quick to learn new ways of working).

Attention needs to be paid to management of the process. The plan provides a model for what is expected to happen, but plans usually become out of date very quickly. We know whether we are on track or not if we monitor the process. Monitoring involves collecting information about whether targets have been met as planned. If some targets have not been met, plans have to be revised and there are often implications for the later stages of change if delays are caused in the early stages. Regular reviews enable people to take an overview of progress and to discuss any changes to the plans. It is often helpful if the reviews include many of the people progressing the activities and tasks because they will understand and be able to explain to others why there have been difficulties.

Reviews are not only about dealing with problems, they are also about noting success and sharing credit for achievements. It is very encouraging to have some early success to encourage everyone and to increase confidence in being able to make changes successfully. Early 'wins' help to keep up momentum, especially if people enjoy feeling the success. Celebrations are helpful when there is something significant to mark.

'Most people are thermometers that record or register the temperature of majority opinion, not the thermostats that transform and regulate the temperature of society.' (Rev. Martin Luther King, Jr.)

Motivation might be an issue, even if people fully support the direction of change. People who realise that their work is going to change significantly will worry about the impact on their salaries and employability. It is important to keep in touch with the people who are affected by change and to listen to concerns as they emerge. Where there are practical steps that can be taken to reduce anxiety, it is helpful to ensure that these steps are taken.

As one change is put into motion, we also need to remember that other things are happening around us. Other parts of the service or our organisation are not standing still until we finish making our change – there will be other developments and our change might impact on other areas. We need to keep in touch with those developments and try to align the progression of our change with other areas, when appropriate. Those who have the skills to foster dialogue are invaluable in facilitating communication.

We also need to check regularly that we are progressing in the direction that we intend and not losing our vision. It is no good to put in mechanisms to make sure that the wheels on the car keep turning if we don't also check that we are making progress in the right direction!

CHANGING CULTURE

The way in which we do things is an outcome of the culture of an organisation or area of work. A vision that involves working in a different way involves achieving a change of culture. Many of our expectations of work arise from our experience of the culture of an organisation. Cultures are notoriously difficult to change because they cannot be controlled in the way that work can be organised because a culture is not something that an organisation completely owns or develops in a deliberate way. Organisations often talk about needing to change the culture, but the culture is complex and developed as a result of the interactions of people and the history that this creates.

The concept of culture is borrowed from anthropology. Organisational culture involves both the formal ways in which an organisation structures its work and the informal ways in which people carry out that work. A culture has features that distinguish itself from other cultures, including what people wear, the logos and badges used, the language, the routines, the stories about success and failure, the way people interact and how premises look. Such symbols carry meanings and emotions (loyalty, pride, inclusiveness or exclusiveness, care or lack of care, formality and informality) which influence every action within the organisation.

Different functions within the same organisation often have different cultures. In a voluntary organisation, for example, a team of carers might have a very different culture from a team of fundraisers. In a large hospital, there might be a very different culture in the operating theatres from that in the finance department. The culture of an area of work is often closely linked with the nature of the work, though differences in culture are more than simply the differences between types of work. Culture includes the way in which the work is done and the feelings that staff have about their work. It includes all the systems that are the ways of doing things in an organisation or area of work, as well as the ways in which the work is understood or experienced in that setting.

Example 12.1:   Culture and change in health and social care

Gerry Johnson (1989) carried out some research to investigate the importance of culture when organisations are involved in strategic change. He identified various elements that contribute to organisational culture and which influence change. We can consider these elements as they might influence change in health and social care

Power structures
There are formal and invisible power structures. The invisible power structure is the basis for the similarly invisible informal systems that often exist to avoid formal procedures. People who hold informal power are not necessarily those in the most senior positions. For example, a person in a position of power might progress requests for resources more quickly for those who support his or her power than for a person who undermines it. Those holding invisible power can progress or block change.

Organisational structures
Most organisations have a chart or diagram showing how all of its parts relate to each other. Some of these show a hierarchy of boxes that indicate different levels of responsibility. Others show how units and departments are grouped. These diagrams represent the formal structure of work in an organisation, and provide the basis for many of its formal systems. Some parts of the formal structure may have to change to achieve a transformation in the way work is done.

Control systems
These are the formal systems that are used within an organisation to control the flow of resources in order to achieve its objectives. They may include financial systems, personnel systems, quality management systems, information management systems and performance management systems. Each of these may have to be adapted to accommodate new ways of working.

Routines
These are the agreed ways of carrying out work that is repeated frequently. They are designed to ensure that predictable, day-to-day work is carried out as efficiently and effectively as possible. In some organisations, routines are written down as formal procedures; in others, they are accepted and taught to new staff as the 'way things are done here'. Informal routines sometimes develop that seem harmless at first but may become features of the culture

that inhibit high-quality performance if they prevent any change or development in the way that work is done.

Rituals

Rituals are ways of behaving that become a standard that is difficult to change. Ritual behaviour is a way of responding that avoids having to think about the consequences of action. For example, someone whose job includes answering the telephone may develop a ritual response in which he or she automatically passes the caller to another person regardless of what the caller has asked for. Such behaviour may not be very damaging to the organisation, but it fails to focus on the needs of the person who has telephoned. Other rituals can be very destructive: for example, there are rituals in some areas of work that put new staff through a sort of trial which allows experienced staff to laugh at their efforts and only admits them to membership of the team after they have submitted to the indignity.

Myths

Myths influence culture in a slightly different way. Every organisation has stories about itself that influence how staff think about the organisation. Sometimes these are positive: for example, 'This organisation cares about its staff' or 'This organisation is a leader in its field'. Other stories might perpetuate less positive characteristics: for example, 'The procedures in this organisation are Byzantine' or 'You will never be able to do that here'. Stories attain the status of myths by being repeated and taught to new staff as things that they must understand if they are to work within the organisation. Myths can make it difficult for staff to consider alternative ways of working when anyone tries to introduce improvements. One of the most destructive myths is 'You will never be able to change this organisation because it is so set in its ways'.

Symbols

There are symbols in every organisation. Some are formal and indicate status or authority: for example uniforms and the insignia on them. Others are informal, such as the dress codes of different staff teams (perhaps suits for managers and more casual dress for staff who work directly with service users).

All of these elements of culture interact to influence the culture of the organisation in which you work.

It is important to understand both the culture of the whole organisation and that of your part of the organisation if you are to work effectively in harmony with the culture of the wider organisation. Some aspects of culture may act as a barrier to change. For example, if staff in one part of the organisation are competing with those in another, it is unlikely that either group will be looking for opportunities to work together to integrate and improve services. If you understand which features of the culture help to support change and which hinder it, you will be in a good position to influence improvements.

ACTIVITY 12.1

Allow 10 minutes.

Think about the culture in your organisation or area of work. Identify some of the cultural features that might make it difficult to change the ways of working.

Power structures:

Organisational structures:

Control systems:

Routines:

Rituals:

Myths:

Symbols:

There may be features of the culture that prevent the team or the whole organisation from performing as well as possible. For example, there might be myths that are taught to new staff that warn them not to be innovative or try to introduce new ideas because these approaches would not be welcome. A familiar myth is to talk of a senior member of staff as 'a dragon', implying that approaching him or her would be dangerous. You might have noticed a tendency to think about staff and service users from only one point of view – for example, as though everyone was white, male and not elderly. Such a culture would make it very difficult for staff to be sensitive to diverse cultures, values and needs when delivering services in a multi-cultural community.

You may feel that there are some aspects of the culture that are helpful: for example, staff might welcome new team members and be supportive in helping them to learn to work in their new setting. People may be questioning the old myths and legends and wanting to free themselves up to work differently.

It is important to identify the features of organisational culture in your area of work and to understand their impact on ways of working. The next step is to consider whether culture can be changed, and, if so, how this might be achieved.

Gareth Morgan used metaphors as a way of analysing the differences between organisations. He suggested that many organisations could be seen as machines:

> Consider, for example, the mechanical precision with which many of our institutions are expected to operate. Organizational life is often routinized with the precision demanded of clockwork. People are frequently expected to arrive at work at a given time, perform a predetermined set of activities, rest at appointed hours, then resume their tasks until work is over. In many organizations one shift of workers replaces another in methodical fashion so that work can continue uninterrupted twenty-four hours a day, every day of the year. Often the work is very mechanical and repetitive. Anyone who has observed work in the mass-production factory, or in any of the large 'office factories' processing paper forms such as insurance claims, tax returns, or bank checks, will have noticed the machine-like way in which such organizations operate. They are designed like machines, and their employees are, in essence, expected to behave as if they were parts of machines.
>
> (Morgan, 1986, p. 20)

An alternative way of viewing organisations is to think of them as living organisms:

> As we look around the organizational world we begin to see that it is possible to identify different species of organization in different kinds of environment. Just as we find polar bears in arctic regions, camels in deserts, and alligators in swamps, we notice that certain species of organization are better 'adapted' to specific environmental conditions than others. We find that bureaucratic organizations tend to work most effectively in environments that are stable or protected in some way and that very different species are found in more competitive and turbulent regions, such as the environments of high-tech firms in the aerospace or electronics industries.
>
> (Morgan, 1986, p. 39)

Viewing an organisation as an organism helps us to consider it as a part of its environment. This metaphor emphasises that an organisation or area of work has to adapt to ensure that it continues to meet the ever-changing needs and demands of its environment. Another metaphor suggested by Morgan is that organisations can be like brains: they can focus on learning and developing innovative ideas and approaches. This metaphor builds on the previous one of the organisation as an organism, emphasising the need to learn from experience in order to respond to environmental changes and opportunities.

Culture is a strong force and can be a major impediment to change. It is a system of beliefs and a way in which people confer meaning on what they do, which suggests that it is not something that can be easily changed. Beliefs and values just aren't like that. Everything we know about psychology suggests that our beliefs about our work and our fellow-workers are often deeply held, reinforced over time, and hard to change. When they do change, the process is more likely to be a gradual, bit-by-bit affair than a sudden wholesale conversion to a completely new set of beliefs. (Indeed, when we come across someone who changes their 'mind set' very rapidly, we often doubt their reliability and judgement.) Organisational cultures can take a generation or more to build up. It is therefore likely that they will also take an appreciable time to change.

Although it is unrealistic to expect to be able to reshape organisational cultures rapidly, it is possible to influence change. We can encourage discussion of values and attitudes. We can emphasise values such as integrity and trustworthiness. We can challenge behaviour that does not respect service users or their interests. We can demonstrate respect for all staff and provide strong and unequivocal support for equal opportunities policies. We can encourage innovatory thinking and a climate of constructive criticism.

You might consider that the culture of your area of work is not always helpful in supporting staff in their work. People who feel unsupported can become negative and make it difficult for others to work effectively. You can intervene by offering more support and by giving positive feedback wherever it is possible to recognise achievements. A team can often be helped to become more positive by focusing on the experience of service users and looking for ways in which it could be improved. If you can discuss these issues openly with your staff, you will be taking action that will – in a small way at first – affect the culture.

In health and care organisations the range of different cultures brings the benefits of diversity. Diversity offers the opportunity to consider many different perspectives and viewpoints, to develop ways of thinking and working that accommodate diversity.

WORKING WITH RESISTANCE

There are many reasons why people might resist change. Some people simply have a low tolerance to change and will want to reduce their own discomfort. Others might see the change as causing them to lose something that they value, perhaps loss of freedom to work in a particular way that has personally suited them. Some might not be convinced that the proposed change is a good thing for the organisation or for their area of work and others might misunderstand the proposals or lack trust in those who are leading the change.

There are ways of overcoming much of this resistance. Effective communication with careful listening and explanation can reduce misunderstanding. Discussion about the reasons for change and the external pressures for change may help some to understand why it needs to happen. Participation in developing the vision and the direction will often win people over to tolerating the change even if they cannot be enthusiastic. Negotiation over particular issues with individuals and groups may gain further agreement. As a last resort, it might be necessary to accept that the change will not suit everyone and that those who are not willing to move in the direction of the organisation should not be allowed to hold it back. If this decision is necessary, then the implications will usually involve careful and detailed management to agree how the individuals concerned should leave the organisation. This is a difficult decision to make, but if the proposed change is essential to the future of the organisation then there may be no choice about progressing the change and accepting the costs.

Example 12.2: Dealing with conflict

Many people find it difficult to deal with conflict and confrontation. In change situations emotions are often high and conflict can flare up unexpectedly. There are many apparent causes of conflict, but these often involve differences in beliefs, values, assumptions and expectations. Conflict can also arise from misunderstandings, lack of respect for differences and changing relationships. Sometimes people misuse power or authority or are simply unreasonable.

There are some strategies that you can use to manage conflict. If issues are raised that it is useful to discuss, then allowing conflict is better than smothering the issues. Sometimes conflict arises as a result of a temporary set of conditions and it may be more appropriate to offer support and try to smooth ruffled feathers until the conditions improve. In some cases it is possible to anticipate conflict and try to prevent it. We can do this only if we are aware of potential clashes and have the means to avoid direct challenges.

We can often reduce the likelihood of conflict by the ways in which we organise work. Conflict is often the result of situations in which some people see personal gains and others losses. We can agree goals, tasks and activities before work is started to reduce conflict over values, ways of working and roles. Good information and communications help to avoid misunderstandings. Organising and resourcing work carefully reduces the possibility of some feeling overloaded and seeing others working less hard.

Another way of considering conflict is to consider the degree to which people assert their aims to satisfy their own needs and concerns and the degree to which they are prepared to co-operate to meet the needs and concerns of others. Thomas (1975) identified five strategies that can be used to resolve conflict:

- Avoiding – Low levels of both assertion and co-operation allow conflict to rumble on unchallenged. This may lead to one party being allowed to bully another or it may allow the cause of the conflict to become worse, so is unlikely to be a useful strategy.
- Smoothing – This can be achieved if there is enough co-operation and people agree to respect differences.
- Competing – When both parties are assertive but not co-operative, competition leads to winners and losers.
- Collaborating – This is possible when both assertion and co-operation are high and people are prepared to pay close attention to differences.
- Compromise – With moderate degrees of both assertion and co-operation, it might be possible to find common ground and compromise. This often requires people to give something up and so is often less satisfying than co-operation.

There is no single 'best way', but different options that can work in different circumstances.

IDENTIFYING SUPPORT AND RESISTANCE

One of the most useful techniques for identifying where support and resistance lie in relation to a proposed change is the force field diagram. A force field diagram helps you to understand your current situation so that you can make specific plans to work with both support and resistance to the proposed change. When you draw a force field, you identify the forces that are helping to drive your change and those that are opposing it. Having identified the forces, you can then decide which positive forces you can take advantage of and which negative ones you can try to reduce. It is a useful tool to apply to any change project, whether the proposed change is major or minor.

Example 12.3:   Force field analysis

Force field analysis is a tool originally developed by Lewin (1947). It assumes that in any change situation there are two sets of forces, those driving the change and those that oppose or restrain it. These forces can be written on a chart using arrows to indicate their directions and relative strengths (Figure 12.1). It is important to recognise that they are forces as perceived by the people involved in the change. For example, there may be no intention to make staff redundant but if any staff believe that the change will make them redundant, the restraining force exists.

You begin the diagram by writing a clear statement of the change you want to make. You then identify all the forces that support and drive the change down the left side of the chart. On the right side you write all of the forces that resist or restrain the change. As you write each force, put an arrow under the note to show the direction but use the strength of the arrow to indicate the strength of the force. You will produce a diagram with opposing arrows of different widths to show their force. If the driving forces for change are stronger than the restraining forces, progress can be made.

The list of forces can be developed by yourself, but it is usually helpful to do this with others so that different perceptions of the situation can be discussed and included. It can sometimes be useful to cluster them under different headings and to use these headings to prompt ideas. Typical clusters would include:

- *personal* (for example fear of redundancy, loss of competence or loss of pride);
- *interpersonal* (for example A does not talk to B);
- *intergroup* (for example perceived loss of status, or competition for space or equipment);
- *organisational* (for example shortage of resources or new management structures);
- *technological* (for example electronic records have been computerised or new equipment needing new skills);
- *environmental* (for example there are more older people or the law on mental health is amended);
- *cultural* (for example perceived loss of professional status if roles change).

The diagram presents the situation as a summary of the forces that you have identified. You can use it to help you to progress the change by examining each of the forces to think about whether you can do anything to reduce the resisting forces. This is usually the best place to start because if you increase the pressure from the driving forces the resistance is likely to increase. Attempts to force change are often unsuccessful because of strong resistance.

There are some approaches that you might take to reduce resistance:

- increase communication about the better future described in the vision and interpret it for those with particular concerns to reassure and, if necessary, incorporate amendments that would reduce their worries;
- emphasise the common values that underpin the vision and direction;
- emphasise the benefits that would be produced for everyone, particularly the benefits for service users;
- discuss specific fears and worries to correct misunderstandings and reduce anxiety;
- identify those who have particular influence and respect and ask them to demonstrate their support for the change.

The force field may have identified some resisting forces that include significant individuals whose influence is strong and could be very damaging if they do not support the change. There is a technique that you can use to assess the strength of support offered by the key individuals involved in the change. Once you have clarified who will help you to progress the change and whose resistance will present obstacles, you can consider what can be done to reduce the power of those who are resisting.

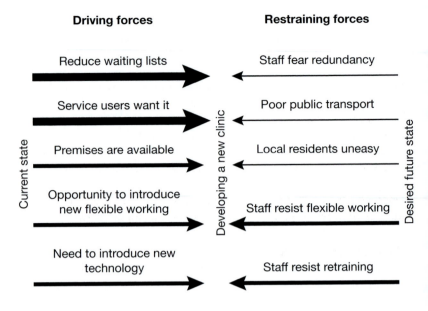

Figure 12.1   Driving and restraining forces

COMMITMENT PLANNING

The aim of commitment planning is to examine how you can build a critical mass of supporters. A commitment plan is a chart in which the key people or groups are listed down one side of a sheet of paper. Across the top are four headings that indicate levels of commitment:

- Opposing – strongly resists the change;
- Allow – will not oppose the initiative but will not actively support it either;
- Help – will support the change with time and other resources, provided someone else will take the lead;
- Make – will lead the change process and make it happen.

Mark each individual or group on the chart with an 'O' to indicate his or her current position. Then put an 'X' to indicate where you would like them to be, thinking in a realistic way about how much they might move. It is unlikely that anyone would move from strong opposition to making the change happen, but if you can influence them to move to a position where they allow progress and withdraw their direct opposition they will be far less of an obstacle. People who are in the 'Allow' position might be moved into becoming helpers if they can be reassured that not too much will be asked of them. The chart will also help you to assess whether there are enough influential people who are committed to leading and making the change happen. If these seem to be too few, you might need to request more support from senior people in the organisation. You might also consider encouraging wider leadership from people at different levels who are enthusiastic about the change and who can influence and inspire others. Also consider involving people outside your immediate work area or organisation. Service users or representatives of service user groups may be pleased to help you. Staff in agencies whose services link with yours may also be able to offer support.

Once you have identified whose commitment is needed, there are a number of ways of gaining it. Here are some suggestions:

- Find out what aspects of the change are unacceptable to the person whose commitment you need, then try to address the specific problems or help these people to solve the problems themselves.
- Find out more about the problems in ways which do not threaten people or force them to adopt stances. For example, hold a private unstructured meeting to talk around a problem, with no minutes taken and with no outcomes other than a better understanding of the issues.
- Use educational and learning settings to encourage open cross-boundary debates and encourage individuals to find opportunities in the change for personal development.
- Be a role model – as a leader, behave in ways that are in keeping with the desired change.
- Use the influence of respected colleagues and peers. This can be particularly helpful in professional cultures.
- Encourage sharing – expose people to others' successes in ways that enable them to copy useful ideas.
- Encourage discussion – demonstrate that there are different views of the situation and the potential opportunities and that people involved see the change in different ways.
- Trade – 'Do this for me, and I will do that for you.'
- Use any power you have to reward desirable behaviour; ignore or punish inappropriate actions.

There is a balance of forces in any change situation, and reducing constraints is frequently more effective than increasing pressure. Change requires a critical mass of supporters and it is important to build this commitment.

In this chapter we have considered both how to inspire others to take action and also how to maintain morale when spirits are flagging. Culture change is acknowledged to be difficult and slow to

Nelson Mandela commented on his relationship with de Klerk: 'He had the foresight to understand and accept that all the people of South Africa must, through negotiations and as equal participants in the process, together determine what they want to make of their future. . . . I never sought to undermine Mr de Klerk, for the practical reason that the weaker he was, the weaker the negotiations process. To make peace with an enemy, one must work with that enemy, and that enemy becomes your partner.' (Mandela, 1994, pp.734–735)

achieve. It is likely to need considerable support from within a culture to change the ways in which people work. Once a change is under way, there are likely to be conflicts to resolve. We concluded the chapter by reviewing some ideas about how conflict might be approached.

CHAPTER 13

REVIEWING, REVISING AND REFLECTING

This chapter brings us to the last stage in the leadership process: reviewing, revising and reflecting. These activities have aspects of both looking back and looking forwards. We look back to see what has worked as intended and what has not. In looking back to review what has happened against the plan, we can also try to learn from events.

First we consider the extent to which the intended change has been achieved. We can do this by reviewing the change that has been achieved against the plan. If there is a discrepancy, there are two options: we can either revise our plans to try to bring our activities back into line with our original plan or we can revise the plan to incorporate a change of timing, costs or quality. We explore how we can ensure that a cycle of change is completed and has stability and how we 're-freeze' the organisation so that the conditions that we have created during change become the new accepted normal state.

We then look at how we can evaluate the change process. This involves both reviewing the change process against the criteria we set for success and reviewing the extent to which it has achieved our vision. We also discuss the ways in which learning can be gained from this experience for individuals, teams and the organisation.

We then review our new position, the new normal state that the change process has achieved. This may have completed a cycle of change and may allow time to pause and reflect, or it may have revealed other urgent issues to address. This brings us to a review of the process of leading change in health and social care services and the central concern about improving services for the service user.

REVIEWING AND REVISING

We use plans to help us to organise and schedule the activities and tasks that will progress the change. Plans, however, are a rather abstract way of representing the ideal process and change rarely fits the ideal conditions. As the actual progress is monitored and compared with the intentions in the plan, there are usually many variations. There are also many reasons for the differences as people try to overcome difficulties and sometimes take longer than was estimated to complete tasks. Sometimes materials or equipment are not available when required and delays are caused. Sometimes tasks are completed more quickly than was planned. A plan is only an estimate.

If the plan is to continue to be useful as events move at a different pace from the schedule, it needs to be revised. It is not wrong to change a plan – it is the only way to manage change in a flexible and practical way. If you regularly review what progress is made against the targets that were set, you are in a position to consider the implications and revise the plan accordingly. This is why it is so important to set targets and to monitor progress. These activities all contribute to understanding what is happening and maintaining some control over progress. Delays can be costly if a number of people are involved and if other resources have been ordered in expectation that work could be carried out on particular dates. If the plan can be revised in time, the work can be rescheduled to make better use of time, resources and energy. This is also important as it signals that the original plan is not the measure of success but only a tool to help to manage progress towards the achievement of the objectives that really matter. If people begin to think that they are failing but could do nothing to avoid the failures, they will soon feel demoralised and progress will become more difficult.

As progress nears completion of the planned change, some attention can be paid to how to signal that the process is finished. Ideally, all the objectives will be achieved and success can be celebrated. It is important to recognise this stage, because sometimes people work very hard to achieve a change but in the final stages of moving into the new ways of working we forget to mark the achievement. It is often helpful to take a brief look backwards to remind everyone how far they have moved.

We have discussed management of change as though it can be controlled by setting clear objectives, monitoring, reviewing and revising. This is something of an illusion, because of the complexity of the context in which change happens. These techniques can help us to be aware of the extent to which we are making progress as planned and can allow us to review and revise the plans. We need enough equilibrium to enable people to work confidently but not so much that it stifles innovation. Even when we accept that plans can only be temporary, there is a danger in thinking that change can be controlled. If we focus too much on the mechanisms of control, we stifle creativity and suspend discussion of alternatives as new possibilities become apparent.

A better way may be to progress through self-awareness and modification of thinking and acting in response to environmental factors. This approach also has its dangers, mainly in our difficulty in becoming sufficiently aware. Some would say that our traditional knowledge about the inter-connectedness of everything has been forgotten and we have made false divisions between work and family, body and soul, animate and inanimate worlds, men and women, animals and people. We have put a value on being busy that makes it more difficult to take time to think and reflect. Time has become a problem more than a benefit and levels of stress are high. Modern feelings of alienation are encouraging many people to reconsider the balance of work and other aspects of their lives. Change is a natural process, but somehow we often create stress and tension in the ways that we do things that seem to make it harder than it ought to be.

MAKING CHANGE STICK

It is not always easy (or desirable) to bring a sense of closure to the change process because if people are beginning to work differently, there will probably be many new issues arising that will need continuing attention and adjustment. This type of continuous change is not the same as a planned change that makes a significant difference to the ways in which people think and work. In the 're-freezing' stage of change, the new ways of working need to become the new routine processes. The change will be embedded only if the new ways align with the culture or cultures in the area of work. Sometimes new processes have to be carefully linked with existing ones that have not been part of the change. If any links had been overlooked in the initial planning, they will soon become apparent as gaps in the service. Gaps in the service are more likely to demonstrate an unsuccessful change than a successful one, at least for those who are inconvenienced.

The change cannot be considered to be successfully completed until the systems that are involved are all running smoothly and without interruptions and gaps. The transformation process that changes inputs into outputs should be working better than before the change. Many will ask whether the change has been successful and an evaluation is often required.

EVALUATION

Evaluation involves making a judgement about value. If it is to be effective, evaluation needs to be focused in some way so that it is clear what is to be judged and what the considerations are likely to be. Evaluations are often held to report on the value of outcomes achieved in relation to the investment of resources to achieve that outcome. Where value is concerned, opinions often vary, and one of the key questions to ask at an early stage is who should carry out the evaluation and whose opinions should be taken into account. Evaluations are usually reported in some way and often make recommendations for future change.

An evaluation will often be based on the information gained through monitoring during the change process. This will attempt to identify:

- whether the objectives have all been achieved;
- which aspects of the process went well;
- which aspects went less well;
- what you would do differently next time.

The aim of this type of evaluation is to understand the reasons for success or failure and thus to learn from the experience in order to improve on performance in the future. At the end of a planned process it is possible to evaluate the extent to which each stage of the change went to plan. It is also possible to explore the implications of any deviations from the original plan. This might reveal that planning could have been more detailed or accurate, that there were obstacles that had not been predicted, that estimates had been inaccurate or that other aspects of the relationship between plans and actions could have been managed more effectively.

A broader evaluation might consider the extent to which the change succeeded in achieving its purpose as a contribution to the progress of the service or organisation. This type of evaluation might be wide enough to include all recent change within an area of work to investigate whether the contributions made by each were good value. It might also consider whether the value could have been increased by managing them in a different way, perhaps by linking them into a large formal project or by splitting them into smaller projects. Although it will be too late to change what has happened, much can be learnt that can inform how future change is defined and managed. For example, it might be found that more assistance is needed to enable managers to estimate costs and times and that other resources from the organisation (perhaps finance, personnel or health and safety) could have helped. The lessons learnt from evaluations can be used to inform higher-level strategic planning.

DESIGNING AND PLANNING AN EVALUATION

A formal evaluation can be both time-consuming and expensive because of the numbers of people involved and therefore must be carefully designed and planned. The following questions will help you to begin to plan:

- What is the evaluation for?
- Who wants the evaluation?
- What is to be evaluated?
- What information will be needed?
- How and from what sources will the information be gathered?
- How will criteria for evaluation be set and by whom?

- Who will do the evaluation?
- Who will manage the process?
- How will the findings be presented?
- What use will be made of the findings?

All of these questions relate to the overall purpose in deciding to hold an evaluation and if each is considered as part of the design process, the answers will enable the process to be planned.

The purpose of the evaluation should be considered in order to identify clear aims and objectives for the process. It is helpful to decide where the boundaries of the evaluation should lie – how much or how little is to be evaluated? A cost is involved in collecting information and preparing documentation as well as in holding the necessary meetings. You might save some expense by considering the extent to which already existing information might be used. The purpose of an evaluation also determines, to some extent, who the audience for delivery of the results should be. The nature of the audience may also determine the way in which the results of the evaluation are reported and used.

A formal evaluation of a collaborative project might be held by a group of the key stakeholders, each able to report back to their own group or organisation. It is important that those conducting the evaluation should be able to understand the context and the issues that were raised in the project, but it is also important to try to find people who can be open and objective. This may mean seeking evaluators who did not have any direct role in the processes or outcomes of the project, but who know and understand your organisation well. In some projects in health and social care settings the choice of those who should be involved is constrained by need for confidentiality. Although it is very important to bring a wide range of perspectives into the evaluation, it is not always appropriate for confidential information to be shared outside the small group that would normally need to access it.

Value judgements are relative and subjective and it can be very helpful to have some explicit standard against which judgements can be made. When there are quality standards for any of the outcomes, these provide a framework that can be used, perhaps alongside targets for time-scales and resource use in achieving the necessary level of quality. Another source of comparable data might be found in benchmarks where these exist for similar activities.

Some of the key questions to consider in carrying out an evaluation of the planning and implementation of change are:

- Were all the objectives achieved?
- What went well and why?
- What hindered progress?
- What was helpful about the plan?
- What was unhelpful about the plan or hindered the work?

- Did we accurately predict the major risks and did the contingency plans work?
- Was the quality maintained at an appropriate level?
- Was the budget managed well and did we complete the change within the budget?
- Was the timing managed well and did we complete the change within the time-scale?
- Did anyone or any other departments hinder the change activities?

To address these questions, you will need information from a wide range of sources. If you plan to carry out this type of evaluation, it is helpful to make a plan to ensure that you collect the appropriate data when they become available, rather than expecting to find that they are still all available at the end of the project. In particular, it is usually worth recording the comments and decisions made in review meetings and in any meetings held to resolve problems that are encountered.

A number of methods can be used to collect and analyse data. For example, records kept for monitoring purposes may be used to make comparisons between activities. Records of meetings and other formal events may also provide useful data relating to the sequence of decisions made and issues discussed. Other data might be collected purely for the purposes of the evaluation. For example, interviews or questionnaires might be used to collect a number of different views or focus groups might be used to explore issues with a group of people together. Observation or role-play might be useful if information is needed about how activities are carried out. The balance between qualitative and quantitative data is important because each can supplement the other and it is difficult to achieve an overall picture if only one type of data is used.

When you are planning the data collection for an evaluation, it is usual to try to obtain a range of different types of data. If only quantitative data were available you would only have information about things that could be counted. Although this is often very important, you would have no information about whether quality standards and other expectations had been achieved. The methods you choose to collect information will be influenced by the availability of resources. However, the key things to take into account are:

- the *cost* of obtaining the information in relation to its contribution to the evaluation;
- the *number of sources* from which information should be obtained if sufficient viewpoints are to be represented to ensure that the results are credible;
- the *time* it will take to obtain and analyse the information;
- the *reliability* of the information obtained;
- the *political* aspects of the process – for example, some ways of gathering information may help build up support for the evaluation.

Direct contact with those involved in the project might be the only way in which sufficient information can be obtained to make the evaluation of value.

ANALYSING AND REPORTING THE RESULTS

When planning what data to use in the evaluation it is helpful to consider how the data will be analysed. Usually, there are considerable amounts of data and they may be in several different forms. If you have set clear objectives, it should be possible to identify the data that are relevant in considering each issue. It is usual to consider:

■ quantity, for example how much has been achieved at what cost;
■ quality, was the quality appropriate and not too high or low;
■ what evidence supports claims to quantity and quality;
■ how do the outcomes compare with alternative ways in which similar outcomes might have been achieved;
■ and can anything be learnt from patterns in the evidence that can inform future change.

It can be very time-consuming to analyse data from interviews and observations, but these approaches often collect very relevant data. It is usually the responsibility of the manager of the evaluation to identify the number and types of reports that are required and to ensure that they are prepared and presented appropriately.

The evaluation report will often contain recommendations that suggest further actions. These recommendations need to be discussed by those who make strategic plans and further actions may need to be considered. There may be recommendations that relate to processes and procedures within the organisation. The evaluation may have identified areas that need to change within organisations if they are to be able to operate flexibly to respond to external change.

'It is important that the leadership of the company be, and is seen to be, involved in the change process. Part of that responsibility is to develop . . . dialogue settings – "communities of practice" – in which people can reflect about their accomplishments, their frustrations, their attitudes, and tell their personal stories in their own words.' (April, Macdonald and Vriesendorp, 2000, p. 75)

LEARNING FROM CHANGE

As well as providing opportunities for individual learning, evaluation and debriefing can be a learning experience for the organisation. This learning can be lost if insufficient time is given to thinking the process through at the end of the planned change. The highlights may stick in your mind but the detail will disappear unless it is documented. People are usually very happy to engage in processes to capture learning, unless their experience has been painful and unresolved. If that is the case, it may be necessary to help those individuals to reach a point at which they can accept the change and then to reflect on their experience to help them to come to terms with it. Individual, team and organisational learning cannot always be separated into neat compartments.

Sometimes the opportunities to learn are greater if the change has been turbulent. We often seek to achieve balance because it feels safer, but instability is often the stimulation for meaningful discussion and fresh thinking. As we know from transformational learning, challenge often provokes significant learning because we discover that there is a different way of seeing things or we find that a position we were comfortable to take is no longer an option.

If you have been considering how learning might be captured from the change process, you may already have been doing so in a variety of ways. You may have asked to what extent you have achieved your aims and objectives. You may also have asked whether the future you had envisaged had proven to be realistic. You will probably be asking whether you have succeeded in building a better future for yourselves and for your service users than the one that might have happened if no changes had been made.

There is much to be learnt at an organisational level from the process, including:

- how ideas were successfully developed;
- how ideas were shared;
- how the ideas became accepted as a vision for the future;
- how other people were brought into a supportive coalition to progress the vision;
- how values were explored;
- how the direction was developed;
- how the change was organised and progressed.

Some of these questions might be answered differently from different perspectives, and these might indicate ways that work in some circumstances and ways that work in others. Comparisons might also be helpful, for example, if one team has been more successful in some tasks than another. Asking why some of these things have happened can also be helpful. Some experiments will have been made, probably not always successful, but something may have been learnt that can be usefully shared. Some may have applied ideas that had worked in other circumstances but found that they were not successful in these conditions. Difficulties may have been overcome in innovative ways that others could learn from.

When changes are intended to improve services for service users, we need to involve service users in learning with us about the extent to which the change represents a real improvement. We also need to explore our learning with colleagues in other service areas and agencies as learning together supports more collaborative working.

Teams can be encouraged to take some time before they disband to reflect together on what has worked well and not so well within the team. A discussion of that nature is a good time to decide what has been learnt that could be helpful to others within the organisation. If new ways of carrying out tasks have been developed, these might be captured in a way that can be a resource for other teams in future.

Individuals will often welcome feedback on their contribution after a period of change. This might be organised to include feedback from various perspectives. If we are to encourage people to work confidently and to offer leadership in change, we need to support development in some ways similar to those we normally use to develop performance. Those who have shown some leadership ability might be invited to take more responsible roles in future initiatives.

As individuals, we can develop skills in learning from experience. Some of the key skills are:

- introspection – we need to recognise how we contribute to situations or problems;
- reflection – we need to make time, distance and awareness to reflect;
- enquiry – we need to ask questions to test our assumptions.

Our behaviour and ways of thinking have grown from how we learnt to react in the past. We need to keep checking that these behaviours are appropriate in the present and as we move into the future.

Some thought might be given to the ways in which learning is captured and shared. Simply providing reports and storing these in databases is useful to a limited extent, but learning about ways of doing things will often be best shared in practical settings. Learning that involves working more openly with differences might be shared only by acting out what has been learnt in different groups and in different settings. In this way we can model what we have learnt, demonstrate it and invite others to develop new learning with us.

Although we can see ways in which organisations can use and value learning, this is rarely achieved to any great extent. Senge (1990) commented:

> It is no accident that most organizations learn poorly. The way they are designed and managed, the way people's jobs are defined, and, most importantly, the way we have all been taught to think and interact (not only in organizations but more broadly) create fundamental learning disabilities. These disabilities operate despite the best efforts of bright, committed people. Often the harder they try to solve problems, the worse the results. What learning does occur takes place despite these learning disabilities – for they pervade all organizations to some degree.
>
> (Senge, 1990, p. 18)

Example 13.1:   Organisational learning disabilities

Peter Senge identified seven learning disabilities that can usually be found to some degree in organisations.

1 'I am my position' – We confuse our jobs with our identities. We focus on our day-to-day tasks rather than the purpose of our work. If we are sure that we are doing our tasks well we find it hard to believe that our contribution may no longer be exactly what is needed for our organisation to achieve its purpose in a changing world.

2 'The enemy is out there' – We like to find something or someone outside ourselves to take the blame when things go wrong. When the consequences of our actions come back to hurt us we only see that they have come from outside, not that they started within.

3 The illusion of taking charge – We can confuse being aggressive with being proactive. If we simply become aggressive as a reaction to some provocation, we are being reactive. True proactiveness comes from understanding how we contribute to our own problems. It is about thinking, not about emotional reaction.

4 Fixation on events – We see life as a series of events and look for causes and implications rather than seeking to understand the pattern of connected events. Short-term thinking stops us noticing the slow long-term changes in the environment that are impacting on us and our organisations.

5 The parable of the boiled frog – The nasty story about how a frog when put into hot water will scramble out, but when put into cool water that is gradually heated will not react but will stay there. It only reacts to sudden change, not to gradual change, although both present threats to survival.

6 The delusion of learning from experience – We have many direct and vivid experiences but we often do not experience the results of our actions. This is particularly true in organisations where staff change jobs frequently.

7 The myth of the management team – Management teams usually try to maintain the appearance of a cohesive team and want to be considered as competent individuals. However, to understand and improve the complex cross-functional issues in an organisation, they will have to engage in long-term thinking, address difficult questions, listen to diversity of views and admit that they have no immediate answers.

In Senge's view these disabilities can be reduced by practicing the five disciplines of a learning organisation:

1 Systems thinking.
2 Developing ourselves.
3 Being aware of the mental models that inform our thinking.
4 Developing shared vision.
5 Developing team learning through dialogue.

(adapted from Senge, 1990)

We can try to develop a climate in which learning is valued. If something goes wrong, we can respond by offering help and support and ensure that something is learnt from the event. We can encourage people to question their own practice, to discuss alternatives, and we can encourage experiments that might help us to find better ways. We can demonstrate that we are always learning and sometimes share that learning with others even if it means admitting to an area of incompetence. Our need to appear competent often inhibits sharing what has recently been learnt, but we can accept that competence is not a 'once and forever' state. We need to know and to be able to do different things as our world changes around us. Lifelong learning is a necessity, not an option.

WHERE ARE WE NOW?

This last stage in the process of leading transformational change (see Figure 8.2) is a time to ask ourselves some key questions. These might include:

- Have we improved services for service users?
- Have we held onto the values that we agreed underpinned this change?
- What are the implications of this change?
- What needs to change next?
- Where do we go from here?

We need to take time to pause and reflect, but in reality, change never stops. As we reflect upon these questions, our awareness is heightened of some of the new urgent issues and new opportunities to build on what is going well. This awareness brings us almost immediately back into the cycle with a new set of priorities.

The organic nature of change has led many to think of it as a continuous process rather than a set of connected events. The process of leading through change might be seen as a continuous process through the cycle of change. We conclude the book with some final thoughts about the nature of transformation.

CHAPTER 14

TRANSFORMING

Throughout this book there has been a sense of old and new, of traditional ways of doing things that are in transition but have not yet been fully replaced with new ways of thinking and acting in leading change. We work in organisations that rely on routine and regulatory processes to deliver complex services. We usually acknowledge that the contribution of people who staff these services, whether the organisations are public, private or voluntary, creates the quality of these services. We talk about valuing staff and respecting differences, but we so often fail to demonstrate this. As leaders in our organisations, we have the opportunity to shape transformation. This may only be possible when the conditions are right. One of the greatest difficulties to overcome is complacency because people have to want change before they will contribute to creating a new future. I wonder how bad things have to get before we face up to the need for transformational change?

South Africa is a country that has considerable experience of transformation. The emphasis of leaders of change in that context has been to find a way forward that acknowledged the history and developed understanding. We often talk of the dangers of a 'blame culture' without exploring what it might mean to replace punishment and retribution with an alternative approach. A member of the new parliament in the Republic of South Africa wrote about the issues that the country faced in developing a process to achieve their vision of reconciliation and reconstruction in pursuit of national unity:

> We were faced with a very critical question: was South Africa going down the road of (retributive) justice or was it seeking reconciliation as it addressed its apartheid legacy: These options at the time were presented as being mutually exclusive. The debate appeared to be centred in two camps: on the one hand, on the victims of violations seeking that alleged crimes be accounted for (avenged) by means of retributive measures; on the other hand, perpetrators seeking impunity by way of a general amnesty.

This approach was not compatible with the manner in which our transition had unfolded. We had to find a formula rooted in the need to achieve a balance between dealing with our past and finding a way forward that was in the best interests of the country as a whole. A win–win situation was called for. . . . The challenge was how to achieve both justice and reconciliation – not just one or the other. To achieve this we had to promote a process of genuine reconciliation in our country within the context of attaining social justice through transforming our country into a united, nonracial, nonsexist, prosperous democracy, based on a human rights culture.

> (de Lange, in Villa-Vicencio and Verwoerd, 2000, p. 23)

De Lange goes on to discuss the difficult balance that had to be obtained to focus on the future through a process that sought understanding rather than vengeance, reparation rather than retaliation and victimisation. A process was developed that included both state prosecution and amnesty to provide a way of restoring the moral worth and equal dignity of all people and social equality rather than victimisation. Desmond Tutu, who led the Truth and Reconciliation Committee, commented that apartheid had infected everyone with a sense that human life doesn't really matter:

we need to remind people that they do matter. And if you believe that you matter, then you are going to find it easier to accept that this other person matters as well. There's been a great deal of self-hatred that we have not faced up to. We need to exorcise our self-hatred.

> (Tutu in Swilling, Annecke and Verwoerd, 2002, p. 14)

We might seek to learn from these ways of thinking as we try to value our differences and demonstrate social justice in our organisational contexts. Some suggestions, again from a South African source, pose some questions that we might consider about leading change in organisations:

- How do we get people to work well together?
- How do we honour and benefit from diversity?
- How do we get teams to work together quickly and efficiently?
- How do we resolve conflicts?
- How do we grow people so that they can add value for their company, their community, their society, and their country?
- Is strategy relevant?
- Are concepts like 'organisational vision' and 'mission' still valid?
- How do we partner with our suppliers, previous competitiors and suppliers, to create more energy, more possibilities?
- What are the enablers of synergy in embarking on strategic partnering?

> (adapted from April, Macdonald and Vriesendorp, 2000, p. 86)

Social, cultural, religious, demographic and political issues need to be understood as the critical, relational inputs and outputs of organisational processes. The new leadership, for example, excels in strategic partnering and recognises that all participants in the system are potential partners.

There are always tensions in our organisations between centralised and localised decision making, hierarchies and 'flatness', tight and loose controls, focused and diffused power – but these newer ideas of leadership focus on liberating people to achieve their potential. New concerns are empowerment, facilitation, collaboration, development and growth. We increasingly recognise the diversity of perceptions, the range of different views that are held about our aims, processes and values. In such diversity, relationships become critical to our ability to develop understanding and agreement about vision and direction. Increasingly we may find that if we focus on developing processes that enable our values to be demonstrated, we will have no need to use many of the traditional strategies that we have described in this book that attempt to create change by controlling the route towards a defined outcome. We will think and lead in more organic ways, focusing on our values and our processes, relating everything that we do to our purposes and the environment in which we work.

REFERENCES

Adair, J. (1983) *Effective Leadership*. London, Pan Books.

Adams, J., Hayes, J. and Hopson, B. (1976) *Transition: Understanding and Managing Personal Change*. London, Basil Blackwell.

Alimo-Metcalfe, B. and Alban-Metcalfe, J. (2002) 'Half the battle'. *Health Service Journal*, 7 March 2002.

April, K., Macdonald, R. and Vriesendorp, S. (2000) *Rethinking Leadership*. Cape Town, University of Cape Town Press.

Argyris, C. and Schon, D. (1978) *Organizational Learning: A Theory of Action Perspective*. Boston, MA, Addison-Wesley.

Belbin, R. M. (1981) *Management Teams*. Oxford, Heinemann.

Blake, R. R. and Mouton, J. S. (1962) 'The managerial grid'. *Advanced Management Office Executive*, Vol. 1, no. 9.

Bohm, D. (1994) *Thought as a System*. London, Routledge.

Buzan, T. (1974, many reprints) *Use your Head*. London, BBC Books.

Carter, R. *et al.* (1984) *Systems, Management and Change*. London, Paul Chapman Publishing/Open University.

Checkland, P. (1981) *Systems Thinking and Systems Practice*, Chichester, Wiley.

Cranwell-Ward, J. (1990) *Thriving on Stress*. London, Routledge.

Cross, P. (1981) *Adults as Learners*. San Francisco, Jossey-Bass.

Dawes, M. *et al.* (1999) *Evidence-based Practice: A Primer for Health Care Professionals*. London, Churchill Livingstone.

dddde Bono, E. (1990) *Lateral Thinking for Management*: A Handbook. London, Penguin Books.

Denzin, N. and Lincoln, Y. (1998) *The Landscape of Qualitative Research*. London, Sage.

Department of Health (2001) *Working Together – Learning Together. A Framework for Lifelong Learning for the NHS*. London, The Stationery Office.

Dixon, N. (2000) 'The insight track'. *People Management*, 17 February 2000.

Easterby-Smith, M., Thorpe, R. and Lowe, A. (1991) *Management Research, an Introduction*. London, Sage.

Edwards, B. (1987) *Drawing on the Right Side of the Brain*. London, Guild Publishing/Souvenir Press.

Fiedler, F. E. (1967) *A Theory of Leadership Effectiveness*. New York, McGraw-Hill.

Garratt, B. (1987) *The Learning Organisation*. London, Fontana Paperbacks.

Gawain, S. (1978) *Creative Visualization*. California, New World Library.

Gleicher, D. (1986) quoted in T. Turrill, *Change and Innovation: A Challenge for the NHS*. London, Institute of Healthcare Management.

Goleman, D. (1996) *Emotional Intelligence*. London, Bloomsbury.

Greenfield, T. (2002) *Research Methods for Postgraduates*. London, Arnold.

Grint, K. (1995) *Management: A Sociological Introduction*. Cambridge, Polity Press.

Grint, K. (ed.) (1997) *Leadership: Classical, Contemporary, and Critical Approaches*. Oxford, Oxford University Press.

Handy, C. (1985) *The Future of Work*. Oxford, Basil Blackwell.

Hersey, P. and Blanchard, K. H. (1988) *Management of Organizational Behaviour*. 5th edn, Englewood Cliffs, NJ, Prentice-Hall.

Honey, P. and Mumford, A. (1986) *Using Your Learning Styles*. Maidenhead, Peter Honey Associates.

Institute for Public Policy Research (1999) *A Good Enough Service: Values, Trade-offs and the NHS*. London, IPPR.

Jarvis, P. (1987) *Adult Learning in the Social Context*. London, Croom Helm.

Johnson, G. (1989) 'Re-thinking incrementalism', in D. Asch and C. Bowman (eds) *Readings in Strategic Management*, pp. 37–56. London, Macmillan.

Kaku, M. (1998) *Visions: How Science Will Revolutionize the Twenty-First Century*. Oxford, Oxford University Press.

Knowles, M. (1978) *The Adult Learner: A Neglected Species*, 2nd edn. Houston, Gulf Publishing.

Kolb, D. A. and Fry, R. (1975) 'Towards an applied theory of experiential learning', in C. L. Cooper (ed.) *Theories of Group Processes*, pp. 33–57. London, John Wiley.

Kotter, J. (1990) *A Force for Change*. London, Free Press.

Kotter, J. P. (1996) *Leading Change*. Boston, Harvard Business School Press.

Lewin, K. (1947) 'Frontiers in group dynamics: Concept, method and reality in social science; social equilibria and social change'. *Human Relations*, Vol. 1, pp. 5–41.

Luther King Jr., Rev M. [n.d.] Quotations from speeches distributed by the Martin Luther King, Jr. Center For Social Change, Atlanta, USA.

Mandela, N. (1994) *Long Walk to Freedom*. London, Abacus.

Martin, V. (2002) *Managing Projects in Health and Social Care*. London, Routledge.

Martin, V. and Henderson, E. (2001) *Managing in Health and Social Care*. London, Routledge.

McGill, I. and Beaty, L. (1992) *Action Learning: A Practitioner's Guide*. London, Kogan Page.

McGregor, D. (1960) *The Human Side of Enterprise*. Maidstone, McGraw-Hill.

Megginson, D. and Pedler, M. (1992) *Self Development*. Maidenhead: McGraw-Hill.

Mezirow, J. (1991) *Transformative Dimensions of Adult Learning*. San Francisco, Jossey Bass.

Morgan, G. (1986) *Images of Organization*. London, Sage Publications.

Nolan Committee (1996) *First Report of the Committee on Standards in Public Life*. London, The Stationery Office.

Pedler, M., Burgoyne, J. and Boydell, T. (1991) *The Learning Company*. Maidenhead, McGraw-Hill.

Pedler, M., Burgoyne, J., Boydell, T. and Welshman, G. (1990) *Self-development in Organisations*. Maidenhead, McGraw-Hill.

Pugh, D. S. and Hickson, D. J. (1989) *Writers on Organizations*. London, Penguin Books.

Reason, P. and Rowan, J. (1981) *Human Inquiry: A Sourcebook of New Paradigm Research*. Chichester, Wiley.

Rogers, C. R. (1969) *Freedom to Learn*. Columbus, Ohio, Charles E. Merrill Publishing.

Sang, B. (1999) 'The customer is sometimes right'. *Health Service Journal*, 19 August, pp. 22–23.

Senge, P. M. (1990) *The Fifth Discipline* (reprint 1992). London, Century Business, Random House.

Stringer, E. (1996) *Action Research*. London, Sage.

Swilling, M., Annecke, E. and Verwoerd, W. (2002) 'Path of forgiveness'. *Resurgence*, September/October, No. 214, pp. 14–16.

Tannenbaum, R. and Schmidt, W. H. (1958) 'How to choose a leadership pattern'. *Harvard Business Review*.

Thomas, K. (1975) 'Conflict and conflict management', in M. D. Dunette (ed.) *Handbook of Industrial and Organizational Psychology*. Rand McNally.

Tuckman, B. and Jensen, M. (1977) 'Stages of small group development revisited'. *Groups and Organization Studies*, Vol. 2, pp. 419–427.

van Maurik, J. (2001) *Writers on Leadership*. London, Penguin Books.

Villa-Vicencio, C. and Verwoerd, W. (2000) *Looking Back Reaching Forward: Reflections on the Truth and Reconciliation Commission of South Africa*. University of Cape Town Press; London, Zed Books.

Wedderburn Tate, C. (1999) *Leadership in Nursing*. London, Harcourt Publishers.

West, M. (2002) 'The HR factor'. *Health Management*, August 2002, London, Institute of Healthcare Management. This research is reported more fully in 'A matter of life and death', *People Management*, 21 February, 2002, London, Chartered Institute of Personnel and Development.

Wooldridge, E. and Wallace, L. (2002) 'Modern times'. *People Management*, 4 April, 2002.

Yin, R. K. (1994) *Case Study Research*. London. Sage.

INDEX

accountability 136–7
Adair, John 16; three focal areas of leadership 21–2, 22
Adams, J. 5
age: increasing life expectancy 8
aims and goals: defining 141–2; and learning 44, 47; process of change 11–12; in uncertain conditions 146–8 *see also* vision
Alban-Metcalf, Robert 23
Alimo-Metcalf, Beverly 23
approachability 23
April, K. 55, 81, 96, 171, 177
Argyris, C. 30–1, 89
authority: X and Y styles 20
awareness: of changes 95; defined 95, 96; of drivers of change 96–101; process of change 11–12; self- 64, 96

Bareham, Jon 49
Beaty, L. 49
Belbin, R. M.: teams 74–5
Bennis, Warren 22–3
Blake, R. R.: style grid *18*, 18–19
Blanchard, K. H. 21
Bohm, D. 29
Boydell, T. 89, 142
brain: left and right 36
Burgoyne, J. 89, 142
Buzan, Tony: mindmapping 36

Carter 113
change: awareness of 95; challenging existing practices 34; and choices 101–2; developing agents for 75–9; drivers of 96–101; evaluating 167–71; from external environment 98–100;

force field analysis 160–1; identifying areas for 115–21; incremental 103; individual fear of 5; learning from 5–7, *6*, 171–5; living with 3–4; making it stick 167; messes *versus* difficulties 112–15, *114*; models of 104–8; need for leaders 3, 4–5; organisational 10–11, 102–3, 153–8; planning 140–5; processes and methods of 142–3; resistance and support 158–62; scale of 103; step 103; transformational 103, 108–10, 130, 176–8; transitions 134, 152
charisma: transformational leaders 23
Checkland, P. 115
citizens, demands of 8
Cochrane Library of Systematic Reviews 87
colleagues: and learning 44, 47 *see also* teamwork
commitment: to visions 131–2
communication 161; commitment planning 163; competence in 53, 54; at distance 91–2; listening 126; of planning 148–9; sharing visions 132; transformational leaders 23
competence: concept and qualities of 53–6
conflict: emotional intelligence 64; group relationships 67–8; strategies to resolve 159–60; working with resistance 158–60
consultation 142; within institutions 9
contingency theories 21–2